A Colour Atlas of

AIDS

in the

TROPICS

A Colour Atlas of
AIDS
in the
TROPICS

M A Ansary
PhD, ABIPP, AIMBI
ARPS

Head, Medical Illustration Department
University Teaching Hospital
School of Medicine
University of Zambia, Lusaka.

S K Hira
MBBS, Dip Derm &
Ven, Dip Ven

Consultant Dermatologist
Head, Dermato-Venereology Department
Honorary Lecturer, School of Medicine
Manager, National STD Control Programme
University Teaching Hospital, Lusaka.

A C Bayley
OBE, MBBChir,
FRCS (E), FRCS (Ed)

Associate Professor of Surgery
University Teaching Hospital
School of Medicine
University of Zambia, Lusaka.

C Chintu
MD, FRCP (C),
Dip Amer Board of Paed

Professor of Paediatrics & Child Health
University Teaching Hospital
School of Medicine
University of Zambia, Lusaka.

S L Nyaywa
MD, MPH

Deputy Director of Medical Services
Chairman, National AIDS Surveillance
Committee,
Ministry of Health, Lusaka.

Wolfe Medical Publications Ltd.

To our patients and colleagues

Copyright © M.A. Ansary, S.K. Hira, A.C. Bayley, C. Chintu, S.L. Nyaywa, 1989
Published by Wolfe Medical Publications Ltd, 1989
Printed by W.S. Cowell Ltd, Ipswich, England
ISBN 0 7234 1567 6

A CIP catalogue record for this book is available from the British Library.

This book is one of the titles in the series of Wolfe Medical Atlases, a series
that brings together the world's largest systematic published collection of
diagnostic colour photographs.

For a full list of Atlases in the series, plus forthcoming titles and details
of our surgical, dental and veterinary Atlases, please write to Wolfe Medical
Publications Ltd, Brook House, 2-16 Torrington Place, London, WC1E 7LT,
England.

Contents

Acknowledgements   6
Foreword   7

PART I AIDS in the Tropics

Section 1: History   8

Section 2: Virology & immunology   9

Section 3: Serology   11

Section 4: Epidemiology of AIDS in the tropics   13

PART II Early Clinical Manifestations & AIDS

Section 5: Spectrum of HIV-related disease
Definition of AIDS   14

Section 6: Persistent generalised lymphadenopathy   16

Section 7: Sexually transmitted diseases   18

Section 8: Cutaneous manifestations   28

Section 9: AIDS-related complex (ARC)   55

Section 10: Kaposi's sarcoma   58

Section 11: SLIM disease   88

Section 12: Pulmonary manifestations   91

Section 13: Sepsis   96

Section 14: Diseases of the nervous system   106

Section 15: Other tumours   107

Section 16: Paediatric AIDS   107

PART III Prevention and Health Education

Section 17: Recognised risk groups   117

Section 18: Education for prevention   117

Section 19: Protection of health workers   119

Section 20: Counselling   122

Acknowledgements

Our special thanks to Professor Peter L. Perine, Director of Tropical Public Health, Uniformed Services University of the Health Sciences, Bethesda, USA, who was the driving force behind us from the very beginning until the day we went to our publisher.

We express our gratitude to the following colleagues for their help, encouragement and advice:

Mr. D. Watters, J. Kamanga, Dr. N.P. Luo, Dr. A.H. Kombe, Dr. W.P. Howlett, Dr. G. J. Bhat, Dr. C. Conlon, Dr. B. Bisseru, D. Zulu, P. Chomba and B. Chipanta.

We acknowledge the support given to us by:

National AIDS Surveillance Committee, Ministry of Health, Lusaka.

Prof. K. Mukelabai, Dean, School of Medicine, University of Zambia, Lusaka.

Health Education Unit, Ministry of Health, Lusaka.

Finally, we express our sincere gratitude to our publishers.

Foreword

Infection with the human immunodeficiency viruses (HIV) and AIDS represents a major challenge to health workers around the world. As of 1st July 1988, 100,410 AIDS cases had been reported to the World Health Organization from 138 countries around the world. An estimated 5 to 10 million persons worldwide are currently infected with HIV. Without a specific means to prevent their developing AIDS, the toll of AIDS cases will rise precipitously during the next five to ten years.

Health workers are called upon for many tasks in the face of HIV infection and AIDS. They must diagnose HIV infection and HIV-related illnesses and ensure that HIV is not inadvertently spread through health-care procedures. The community looks to health workers for guidance, for information and education. Health workers must deal with complex psychological, social, legal and ethical issues associated with HIV-testing. Health workers are asked to contribute, through personal and community leadership, to forming an enlightened public opinion.

Within all the other complex challenges of HIV/AIDS, the capacity to diagnose is fundamental to the care and management of HIV-infected persons including those with HIV-related illness. It has been recently said (as it was once said of syphilis) that whoever understands the clinical manifestations of HIV infection will understand all medicine.

This colour atlas of the many manifestations of AIDS observed among patients in the tropics provides useful information to the clinician. While the specific opportunistic infections and malignancies associated with HIV infection will vary in different areas, the lessons to be learned from careful study of this atlas will certainly be useful to clinicians in many parts of the world.

Jonathan M. Mann, MD, MPH
Director, Global Programme on AIDS
World Health Organization
Geneva, Switzerland

Part 1   AIDS in the Tropics
Section 1: History

The acquired immunodeficiency syndrome (AIDS) epidemic was first reported in New York and California in 1981, in previously healthy male homosexuals who presented with opportunistic infections and Kaposi's sarcoma. The term AIDS was officially adopted in 1982. The causative retrovirus, called Lymphadenopathy-Associated Virus (LAV), was identified first in 1983 by Montagnier and colleagues in Paris.

Simultaneously, Gallo and colleagues reported isolation from patients of a virus which they called Human T-cell Lymphotropic Virus type III (HTLV-III). Investigations confirmed the identity of LAV and HTLV-III. By international agreement this virus is referred to now as the Human Immunodeficiency Virus type I (HIV-I).

AIDS was reported in tropical Africa from 1982 onwards while the first (retrospectively recognised) cases in the Americas occurred in 1979. There has been a marked increase in the number of cases reported to the World Health Organisation over the years.

Transmission of AIDS in Africa is primarily through heterosexual activity, whereas in America and Europe the main modes of transmission are sexual contact between homosexuals and bisexuals, and sharing of contaminated needles among intravenous drug abusers.

1

Year	1979	1980	1981	1982	1983	1984	1985	1986	1987	Total
*Africa				3	4	9	20	1033	2627	3696
America	14	56	264	1032	3134	5989	10424	8336	34195	63468
Asia		1		1	8	4	24	30	103	171
Europe		1	6	42	235	536	1326	1542	4559	8253
Oceania				1	6	44	123	170	404	748
Total	14	58	270	1084	3387	6582	11917	11111	41888	75588

*There seems to be under-reporting of AIDS cases in Africa.

1   Table showing the number of AIDS cases by continent reported to the WHO.

Section 2: Virology & Immunology

Human Immunodeficiency Virus (HIV-I)

The acquired immunodeficiency syndrome (AIDS) was first recognised in 1981. It has been clearly established that the cause of AIDS is a human retrovirus called human immunodeficiency virus - I (HIV-I).

The retroviruses were known long before the emergence of AIDS and HIV-I. Many are RNA - containing tumour viruses which cause sarcomas or leukaemias in a variety of animals and mammary cancers in mice. The human T-lymphotropic virus (HTLV) group of retroviruses includes HTLV-I which causes a T-cell leukaemia in man, a related virus HTLV-II, and HTLV-III which is another name for HIV-I.

HIV-I, however, does not lead directly to tumour production but is a member of the lentivirus subgroup of retroviruses also known as slow viruses because they cause chronic infections, which progress slowly over a period of months to years.

HIV-I is a single stranded RNA virus which replicates by using an unique enzyme, reverse transcriptase, to translate its genomic RNA into a DNA copy. This DNA is then inserted as a provirus into the host cell DNA, where it may remain latent or be copied again into viral RNA to produce new virus particles.

HIV-I infects T-helper lymphocytes (CD4/OKT4/LEU3a) and also cells of the monocyte/macrophage series, including glial cells of the brain. In fact, monocyte/macrophages have been described as the main reservoirs of HIV-I. Because DNA copies of HIV-I are integrated into host cells, the virus persists throughout the entire life of the infected individual and duplicates itself every time the infected cell multiplies.

HIV-I was first discovered by Barre-Sinoussi, Montagnier and colleagues at the Pasteur Institute in 1983. They called their isolate lymphadenopathy-associated virus (LAV). Soon thereafter, in 1984, Robert Gallo and co-workers, in the USA, described the same virus but called it human T-lymphotropic virus-III (HTLV-III). Recently HIV-I has become the proper name, on the recommendation of an International Committee on nomenclature.

In 1985, another retrovirus of the HIV family was isolated from persons living in West Africa. This virus was called LAV-2 by the French, who found it in patients with AIDS or AIDS-related complex (ARC). The same virus was isolated from healthy West African prostitutes by other workers who called it HTLV-IV. It has been isolated also in Europe and America and appears to be more closely related to simian T-lymphotropic virus-III than to HIV-I. Among isolates of HIV-II, some seem to cause AIDS, while others may not. Like HIV-I, HIV-II infects T4 lymphocytes. It induces some antibodies that cross react with HIV-I.

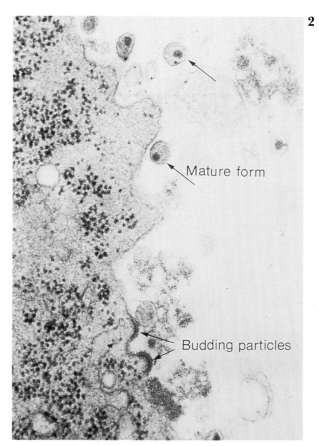

2

2 Human Immunodeficiency Virus (HIV) seen as mature and budding forms in tissue cell line. (By courtesy of R. Gallo et al. Science).

The major proteins of HIV-I are its structural proteins encoded by the **gag** gene which are recognized on Western blots as 15Kd, 17Kd, 24Kd and 55Kd MW bands, the **pol** gene proteins of 64Kd and 53Kd MW, and the **env** gene glycoproteins of 41Kd, 120Kd, and 160Kd MW. The HIV-II virus induces antibodies that cross react with HIV-I **gag** proteins but not with the 41Kd **env** protein.

Remarkable progress has been made in isolating and characterising these presumably new retroviruses within only a few years of the recognition of AIDS. Indeed, nucleotide sequencing of the genomes of many isolates has already been accomplished. Nevertheless, much remains to be learned. Among the unanswered questions are:

How many different viruses can cause AIDS?
What are the co-factors which lead to active disease?

Which are the important immunogens?
Can immunity to these viruses be achieved by vaccination?

Immunology

It has long been known that HIV causes immune dysfunction resulting mainly from depletion of T4 lymphocytes. The T4 cell, among other functions, recognises foreign antigens on infected cells and helps to activate B lymphocytes. The B cell then produces specific antibodies that bind to infected cells and to free organisms bearing the identified antigen, thereby leading to their destruction. The T4 cell also plays a vital role in cell-mediated immunity in killing the infected cells by cytotoxic cells. The T4 cell also influences the activity of monocytes and macrophages which engulf infected cells and foreign particles.

The infection of a T4 cell by HIV begins when a protein, **gp**120, on the viral envelope binds to a protein known as CD4 receptor on the surface of the T4 cell. HIV then merges with the T4 cell and transcribes its RNA genome into double-strand DNA. The viral DNA becomes incorporated into the nucleus of T4 cell and directs the production of new virion particles. These virion particles bud from T4 cell membrane and infect other T4 cells.

The severe depletion of T4 cells seen in patients with AIDS is difficult to explain solely on the basis of destruction of a few infected T4 cells during replication of HIV in them. In the laboratory, other likely mechanisms of T4 cell destruction have been identified: syncytia formation, antiviral activities of cytotoxic antibodies and cells, and cytokines produced by monocytes and macrophages. Syncytia develop after a single infected T4 cell produces **gp**120 on its cell surface and this viral protein has high affinity for CD4 receptors on uninfected T4 cells. Thus, uninfected T4 cells can bind to the infected T4 cell forming a syncytium which cannot function and dies. In the second possible mechanism cytotoxic antibodies and cells destroy any cells which exhibit free viral **gp**120 on their surfaces. Thus, even uninfected T4 cells which have free **gp**120 on their surfaces are susceptible. The third possible mechanism involves cytokines produced by infected monocytes, macrophages and other tissue dendritic cells present in the skin, mucous membranes, liver, spleen and brain.

3 Western blot A test to recognise components of antibody response to HIV.

Blot no.	Reactivity
2,4,5,6,7	Positive
3	Negative
8,10	Faint **gp**41
9	Faint **gp**1 & **p**24

B cell function in HIV disease patients is also impaired. Polyclonal B cell activation has been shown as a major feature of B cell dysfunction. In spite of high levels of antibodies in these patients, the role of these antibodies is not known. Besides B cell, T4 cell and macrophage dysfunction, the natural killer cell activity is also reduced in these patients.

Whatever may be the mechanism of depletion of T4 cells it seriously impairs the ability of the immune system to fight against viruses, fungi, parasites and certain bacteria, including mycobacteria. It is generally recognised that as T4 cell count falls below 400 chronic infections of the skin and mucous membranes set in and as the count falls further, systemic infections appear.

Section 3: Serology

Evidence of HIV-I infection may be gained by isolating the virus, by demonstrating antibodies to it or by detecting viral antigens. Anti-HIV antibodies usually become detectable between three weeks to three months after exposure to HIV-I.

For serological tests, antigen can be prepared from HIV-I grown in cell lines and purified, or prepared synthetically by genetic engineering. The serologic tests which are used for diagnostic purposes are:

Agglutination and ELISA (enzyme-linked immunosorbent assay)
Immunoblotting
Immunofluorescence

ELISAs use an enzyme conjugated to give a colour reaction between specifically bound HIV-I antigen and antibodies to it. Since HIV-I serologic tests were licensed in 1985, they have been used in many countries throughout the world. Although the early tests were sensitive, they were not very specific. Subsequent ELISA tests have been developed which use purified HIV-I virus or genetically engineered HIV-I antigens which have high sensitivity and specificity.

The choice of a serologic test should be based on its availability, cost, specificity, sensitivity, simplicity, and the other possible infections in the environment that may cause cross-reactions.

4 Quantum spectrophotometer II used to read optical density of ELISA test.

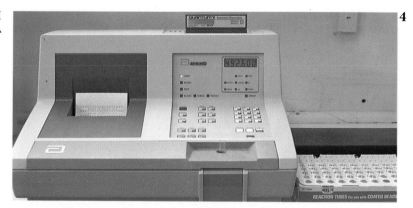

5 Anti-globulin ELISA test for detection of anti-HIV antibodies. Various shades of brown colour indicate a positive test.

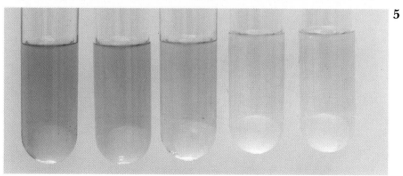

Currently, the most widely used confirmatory tests are the Western blot and ELISA using genetically produced HIV-I antigens.

Detection of various classes of immunoglobulins is also widely used. The IgM anti-HIV response is of particular interest as appearance of IgM slightly precedes the IgG response. Detection of individual immunoglobulin classes is of particular interest in babies, because IgM does not cross the placenta and when present it is made by the baby, whereas IgG from the mother crosses the placenta. Thus IgM anti-HIV antibodies in a young baby might indicate that the baby has been infected, although the tests are not commercially available and methodology is cumbersome. Presence of IgG may only mean that the mother was infected. However, if IgG antibodies persist in the baby past 15 months of age, the baby is infected.

Tests have also been developed to detect HIV-I antigens e.g. HIV core antigen (**p**24). These tests are of particular importance in detecting early infection when HIV-I antibodies are not detectable because they are absent or present in low concentration. Isolation of HIV is very demanding; it requires technical expertise and a sophisticated laboratory so it is seldom used as a diagnostic procedure. Simple tests are being developed for laboratories with inadequate facilities for ELISA or radio-immunoassay.

6

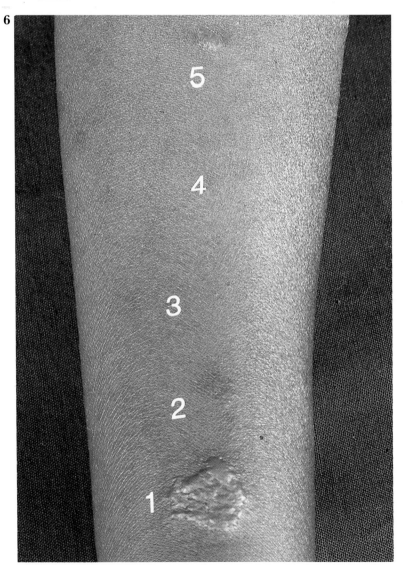

6 Hypersensitivity skin tests

Known antigen	Result
1 - PPD	+
2 - Candidin	−
3 - Trichophytin	−
4 - Tetanus	−
5 - Mumps	−

Section 4: Epidemiology of AIDS in the Tropics

The acquired immunodeficiency syndrome (AIDS) is a relatively new disease in the tropics and has created an urgent public health problem throughout the world. In hospitals of some cities in the tropics, as many as 3-10% of all admissions are due to AIDS or HIV-related disease. This has seriously strained the health budgets of some countries. There is increasing evidence that prevalence of HIV infection in rural areas is much lower than that encountered in urban areas. Most tropical countries are undergoing rapid urbanisation which might influence the future course of the epidemic. The World Health Organisation estimated in 1988 that 5-10 million people might be infected world-wide and 1 million new cases of AIDS will be seen over the next ten years. There is no evidence of racial susceptibility to HIV infection.

Epidemiologic studies indicate that transmission of HIV-I in Africa and Haiti is primarily by heterosexual intercourse as indicated by the 1:1 sex ratio of HIV infections. Between 80 and 90% of those infected are in the most sexually active age group (20-40 years) and have had multiple sexual partners. There has been some evidence that genital ulcer disease might facilitate transmission of HIV.

Other modes of transmission are by blood and blood products (as seen in haemophiliacs), and by congenital or perinatal transmission from mother to child. This has important implications for family size and population structure in the tropics where more than half of infected adults are women of child-bearing age.

Homosexuality and intravenous drug abuse are rarely acknowledged by Africans and these probably are not significant modes of transmission for HIV in Africa. The pattern of HIV-I transmission in the tropical parts of South America, Asia and Oceania has not been established because of the small number of cases that have occurred to date. HIV is not transmitted by casual nonvenereal contact or by blood sucking arthropods. Transmission via infected needles, scarification instruments, infected organ transplants, and artificial insemination is possible, but its extent is not known. Transmission through breast milk seems to have an insignificant role.

Although HIV-II has been identified in Gambia, Guinea Bissau, Senegal and the Ivory Coast, there is no evidence of this virus as yet in East and Central Africa.

Under-reporting of AIDS cases in Africa is common and laboratory confirmation of the diagnosis is not widely available. This makes it difficult to present a clear picture of its epidemiology. However, clinical criteria can be used to diagnose HIV-related disease in Africa (Section 5).

7

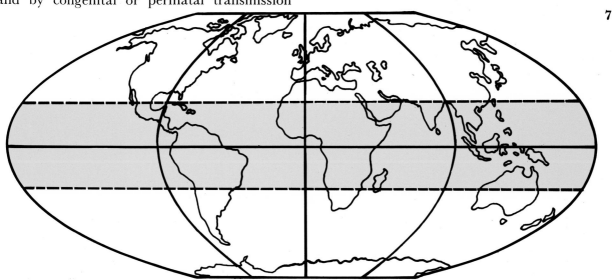

7 Global map showing the tropic band.

Part 2 Early Clinical Manifestations and AIDS

Section 5: Spectrum of HIV-related Disease

Human Immunodeficiency Virus related diseases have a clinical spectrum ranging from asymptomatic infection to the full-blown picture of AIDS. All systems of the body may be affected either singly or in combination. AIDS patients lose the ability to immunologically defend themselves against many infectious agents. Current evidence indicates that progressive immunodeficiency will cause death in most of those infected with HIV-I.

In the northern hemisphere a few patients who acquire HIV infection experience an acute viremic febrile illness, similar to infectious mononucleosus, with or without acute encephalitis, before seroconversion occurs. Such acute-onset illnesses are very rarely recognised in the tropics and possibly misdiagnosed as malaria. However, many patients who appear to have early infections have experienced minor symptoms including lymph node enlargement for several months.

After an incubation period of months or years, HIV-infected persons develop opportunist infections as evidence of deteriorating immune competence. Abnormal neurologic signs may also be detected, although symptoms are uncommon. Once this stage has been reached periods of reasonable well-being alternate with acute or chronic infections. The clinical features are listed below in order of frequency of occurrence and might be as a direct consequence of HIV or due to opportunists/tumours occurring as a result of immunosuppression:

weight loss
persistent generalised lymphadenopathy
chronic cough
recurrent fever
multidermatomal herpes zoster
recurrent diarrhoea
candidiasis
aggressive Kaposi's sarcoma.

There is a slow loss of vitality and weight, with increasingly frequent and serious bouts of illness which interfere with work and social life. This stage may last several years but progresses inexorably to life-threatening infections or tumours which lead to death.

AIDS was defined in 1982 and 1983 by a description of its end-stage diseases. The transition from pre-AIDS to AIDS may be difficult to identify or may depend upon the availability of diagnostic tests. Once progressive disease interferes with a patient's functions in the family and community, return to sustained normal health never occurs. This appears to be the natural history of the disease as seen in the developing and the developed world.

In children the course of the disease is accelerated. In adults intercurrent infections such as tuberculosis and sexually transmitted diseases may precipitate or accelerate the progression of immunodeficiency.

A clinical diagnosis of AIDS is made according to the criteria below. The symptoms and signs of the AIDS-related complex (ARC) are due to a partial loss of cell-mediated immunity. From the available evidence, the progression of the disease is unidirectional from ARC to AIDS. It may be useful in the future to separate the clinical features of the primary HIV infection from symptoms and signs related to opportunistic infections.

CDC/WHO case definition for AIDS, 1988

A case of AIDS is defined as an illness characterised by one or more of the following 'indicator' diseases, with or without laboratory evidence of HIV infection:

1. Without laboratory evidence for HIV infection

If laboratory tests for HIV are not performed or give inconclusive results and the patient has no other cause of immunodeficiency, then any disease listed below indicates AIDS if it is diagnosed by a definitive method.

a. Candidiasis of the oesophagus, trachea, bronchi, or lungs
b. Cryptococcosis, extrapulmonary
c. Cryptosporidiosis with diarrhoea persisting for more than 1 month.
d. Cytomegalovirus disease of an organ other than liver, spleen, or lymph nodes persisting for more than 1 month
e. Herpes simplex virus infection causing a mucocutaneous ulcer that persists for more than 1 month; or bronchitis, pan-pneumonitis, or oesophagitis of any duration
f. Kaposi's sarcoma affecting a patient under 60 years of age
g. Lymphoma of the brain (primary) affecting a patient under 60 years of age
h. Lymphoid interstitial pneumonia and/or pulmonary lymphoid hyperplasia affecting a child under 13 years of age
i. Mycobacterium avium complex or M. Kansasii disease, disseminated (at a site other than or in addition to the lungs, skin, or cervical hilar lymph nodes)
j. Pneumocystis carinii pneumonia
k. Progressive multifocal leucoencephalopathy
l. Toxoplasmosis of the brain affecting a person more than one month of age

2. With laboratory evidence for HIV infection

Regardless of the presence of other causes of immunodeficiency, laboratory evidence of HIV infection together with any disease listed above or below is diagnostic of AIDS.

a. Bacterial infection, multiple or recurrent, including septicaemia, pneumonia and meningitis
b. Disseminated coccidiomycosis

c. HIV encephalopathy
d. Disseminated histoplasmosis
e. Isosporiasis with diarrhoea persisting for more than one month
f. Kaposi's sarcoma at any age
g. Lymphoma of the brain at any age
h. Non-Hodgkin's lymphoma of B-cell or unknown immunological phenotype
i. Any mycobacterial disease caused by mycobacteria other than M. tuberculosis
j. Disease caused by M. tuberculosis, extrapulmonary
k. HIV wasting syndrome ('SLIM' disease)
l. Recurrent septicaemia by nontyphoid Salmonella

Although CDC/WHO case definition is the 'gold standard' for diagnosis of AIDS, the laboratory diagnosis of pathogens in most tropical countries is not possible. Hence, the clinical case-definition used in some African countries might be useful elsewhere in the tropics and is given below:

DEFINITION - Adult AIDS

A case of AIDS in an adult is defined as a patient with no known underlying cause of cellular immunodeficiency who presents with at least two of the major signs associated with at least one minor sign:

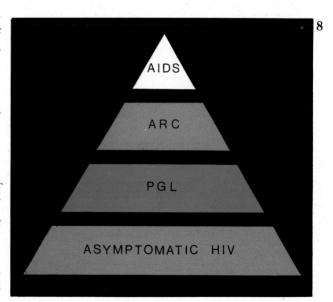

8 Pyramid showing the spectrum of HIV-related disease (courtesy of R.R. Redfield M.D.)

Major signs
weight loss of > 10% of body weight in 1 month
chronic diarrhoea > 1 month
prolonged fever > 1 month (intermittent or constant)

Minor signs
persistent cough > 1 month
generalised lymphadenopathy
herpes zoster
persistent fatigue
night sweats

DEFINITION - Paediatric AIDS

Paediatric AIDS is suspected in an infant or child (under 13 years of age) presenting with at least two major signs associated with at least two minor signs in the absence of known causes of immunodeficiency:

Major signs
recurrent fever > 1 month
recurrent oropharyngeal candidiasis
recurrent pulmonary infections

Minor signs
chronic diarrhoea > 1 month
weight loss or abnormally slow growth
generalised lymphadenopathy
persistent cough > 1 month
extrapulmonary tuberculosis
Pneumocystis carinii pneumonia
confirmed maternal HIV infection

Section 6: Persistent Generalised Lymphadenopathy

Persistent generalised lymphadenopathy caused by HIV is common in the tropics as elsewhere in seropositive persons who are otherwise symptom-free. These enlarged lymph nodes are 1 to 2cm in diameter, discrete, numerous, regular, symmetrical around the sagittal plane and persist for at least 3 months. Usually occipital nodes are noticed first by the patient. Awareness of the enlarged lymph nodes causes anxiety, particularly if they fluctuate in size and cause discomfort. There are no signs of opportunist infections, and haematologic investigations may show no abnormality other than mild lymphopoenia. Oropharyngeal lymphoid tissue commonly becomes hyperplastic to produce tonsillar enlargement comparable to the hypertrophy seen in adolescent children who have recently started school.

When lymph nodes enlarge asymmetrically, or to an average size in excess of 2cm, a biopsy may be indicated to exclude tuberculous adenitis or lymphoma (asymmetrical) or Kaposi's Sarcoma (symmetrical).

Histological examination of persistently enlarged nodes (without secondary pathology) shows marked follicular hyperplasia with an intact network of follicular dendritic cells, increased numbers of macrophages and lymphocytes and in some patients, increased vascularity. As the disease progresses, the lymphadenopathy may disappear. In some cases cytotoxic drugs may precipitate full-blown AIDS with diarrhoea, fever and a variety of opportunistic infections.

Differential diagnoses:

Cervical lymph node enlargement may be due to carcinomas of the head and neck. Nasopharyngeal carcinoma often presents with bilateral deeply fixed nodes in the upper jugular chains, but without symptoms to draw attention to the primary tumour.

Secondary syphilis is an important cause of generalised lymphadenopathy and should be excluded by serologic tests. Infectious mononucleosis and sarcoidosis are both exceptionally rare in Africa, so neither is likely to account for generalised node enlargement.

9 Enlarged posterior cervical and post-auricular lymph nodes in a patient who progressed to AIDS in 2 years.

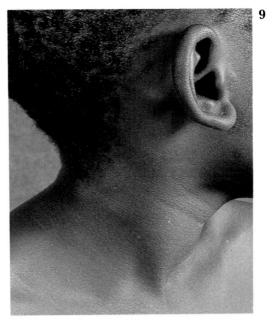

10 Lymph node enlargement in a patient with HIV infection.

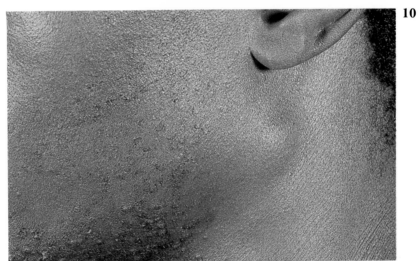

11 Tonsillar hypertrophy in an HIV infected patient with generalised lymphadenopathy.

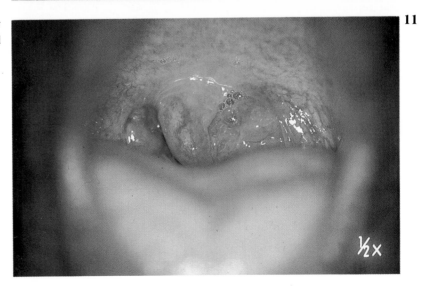

Section 7: Sexually Transmitted Diseases (STDs)

The clinical presentation of conventional sexually transmitted diseases (STDs) occurring in association with HIV disease is often atypical, aggressive and unresponsive to established treatment regimens. As a result, bacterial STDs may require prolonged treatment. In STD practice in the tropics, phagedenic chancroid, suppurative lymphogranuloma venereum, extensive herpes genitalis, recurrent episodes of pelvic inflammatory disease (PID), disseminated molluscum contagiosum, erosive candidiasis, and fulminant growths of condylomata acuminata are encountered with increased frequency. In a study conducted in Lusaka among patients with HIV disease, 50% of male and 73% of female patients had one or more of the conventional STDs when first examined.

Differential diagnoses - STD

The classical presentation of uncomplicated STDs are:

Chancroid

Multiple painful soft bleeding ulcers arising within one week of sexual contact. The inguinal lymph nodes are enlarged, tender and may suppurate.

Herpes genitalis

Multiple small, painful, itchy vesicles lasting for 2-3 weeks. The condition tends to recur.

Lymphogranuloma venereum

The initial genital lesion is small and painless and may be confused with other ulcers. It is later associated with enlarged, painful and firm matted inguinal lymph nodes which can suppurate and form multiple draining sinuses.

Balanitis

Occurs as erosions on the glans penis. It is sometimes associated with subpreputial discharge.

Venereal warts

Multiple filiform or warty growths increasing in size over a period of months.

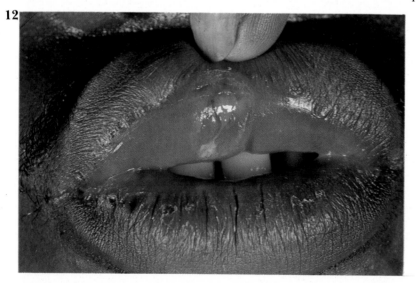

12 17-year-old male presented with an indurated, non-tender, avascular ulcer on upper lip. Investigations revealed motile Treponema pallidum under dark field microscopy. He acknowledged oro-genital sexual contact.

13 This young man with AIDS presented with primary chancre on the shaft of penis (DGI positive) and multiple herpetic lesions on the coronal sulcus and glans. Following treatment with benzathine penicillin, the healing of the chancre was slower compared to non-HIV patients.

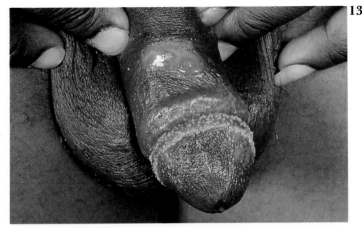
13

14 Relapsing papular and papulosquamous syphilides 4 weeks after adequate penicillin therapy. The patient was HIV positive. The efficacy of syphilotherapy in patients with HIV infection needs further evaluation.

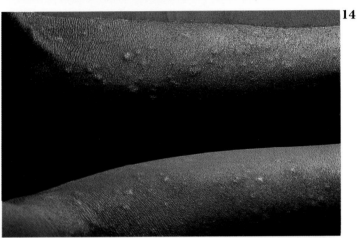
14

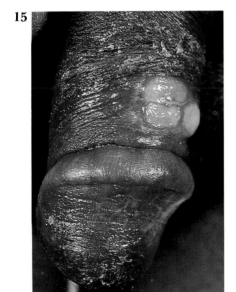
15

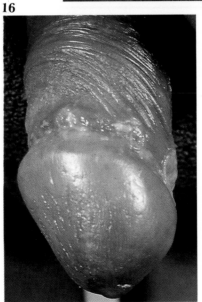
16

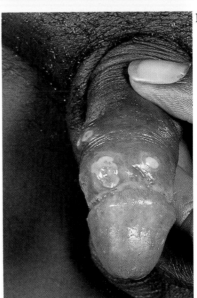
17

15 Classical chancroid showing multiple, superficial, tender ulcers with an erythematous halo.

16 Classical chancroid seen as multiple superficial ulcers in an immunologically normal patient.

17 Classical chancroid.

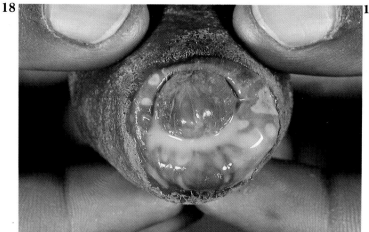

18 Classical chancroid with preputial discharge.

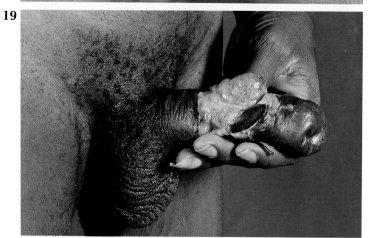

19 & 20 Chancroid often tends to become necrotic in patients with HIV disease. The response to conventional treatment regimens is inadequate.

21 Phagedenic chancroid.

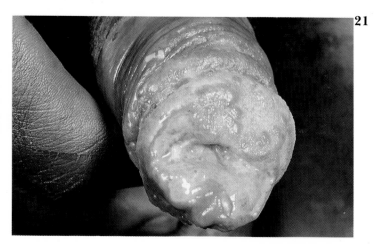

22 Phagedenic chancroid, persistent for two months in a patient with AIDS-related complex.

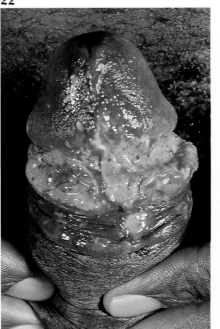

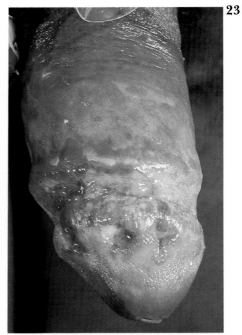

23 Necrotic chancroid in a patient with AIDS.

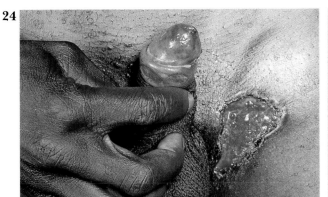

24 HIV-related chancroid unresponsive to therapy.

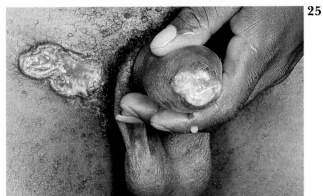

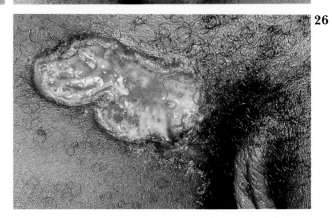

25 & 26 Classical chancroid with multiple superficial ulcers on genitalia and a ruptured bubo. The patient was not infected with HIV.

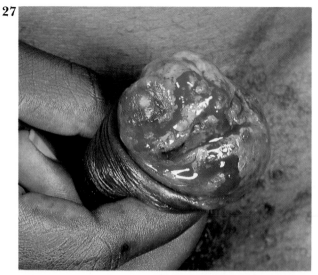

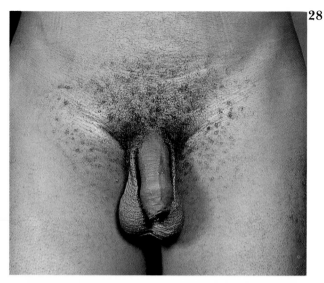

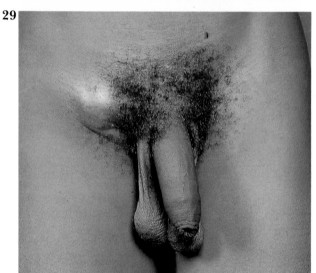

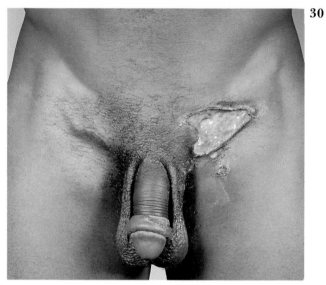

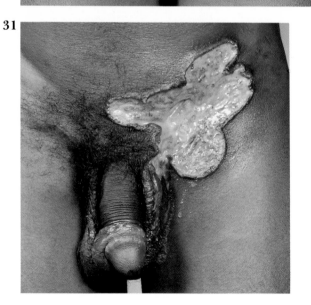

27 Necrotic chancroid in a patient with ARC.

28 Classical lymphogranuloma venereum with "groove" created by the enlargement of the inguinal and femoral lymph nodes which are separated by the inguinal ligament.

29 Classical lymphogranuloma venereum with inguinal bubo. Patient was not infected with HIV.

30 & 31 Superficial ulcers of lymphogranuloma venereum and ruptured bubo in a patient with ARC. Second picture taken 3 months after the patient had received adequate treatment with co-trimoxazole and tetracycline.

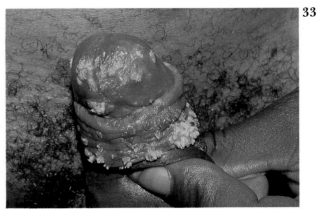

32 **Classical condylomata acuminata** (venereal warts) not related to HIV infection.

33 Florid venereal warts with underlying HIV infection which are often unresponsive to conventional chemotherapy or electro-cautery.

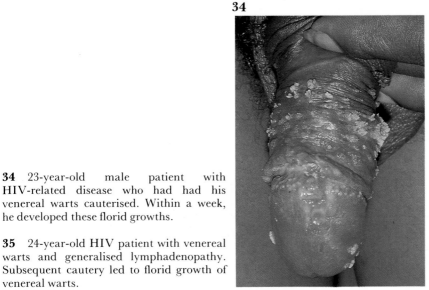

34 23-year-old male patient with HIV-related disease who had had his venereal warts cauterised. Within a week, he developed these florid growths.

35 24-year-old HIV patient with venereal warts and generalised lymphadenopathy. Subsequent cautery led to florid growth of venereal warts.

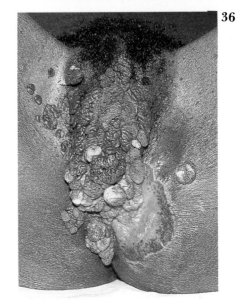

36 This young woman with a history of anaemia had extensive genital warts. Subsequent removal by cautery was followed by growth of fresh lesions. She was found to be infected with HIV.

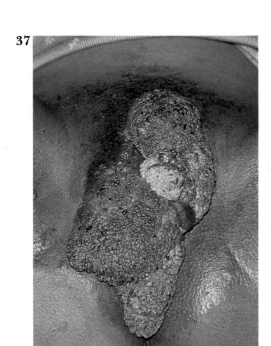

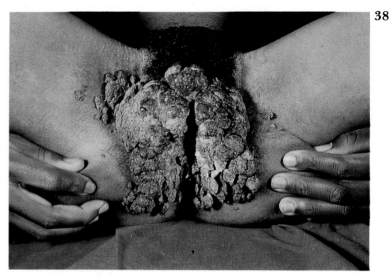

37 & 38 Giant condylomata acuminata in female patients with ARC.

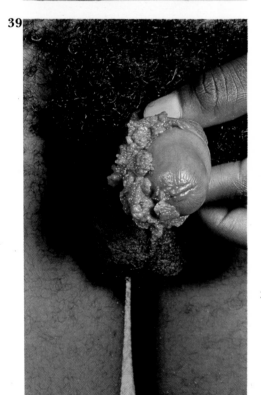

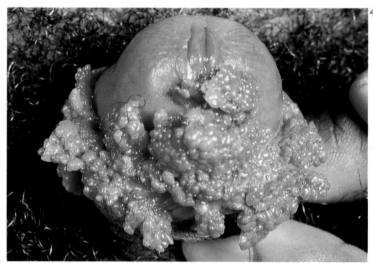

39 & 40 Extensive venereal warts.

41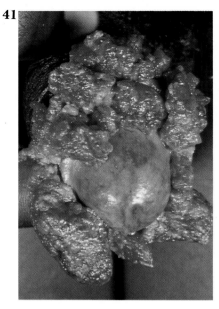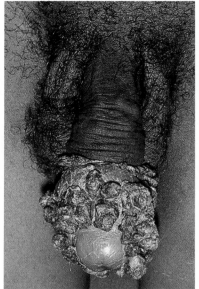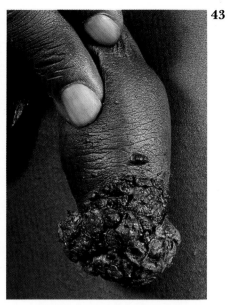

43

41 Extensive venereal warts associated with HIV infection.

42 Fulminant venereal warts in a patient with HIV disease.

43 Extensive venereal warts and genital molluscum contagiosum in a patient with ARC.

44 Extensive venereal warts in a patient with ARC. The lesions proliferated rapidly and did not respond to electro-cautery.

45 Extensive venereal warts on the vaginal wall in a patient with ARC.

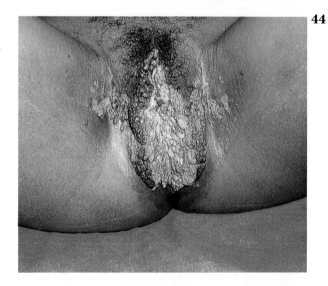

44

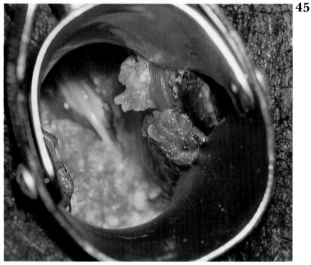

45

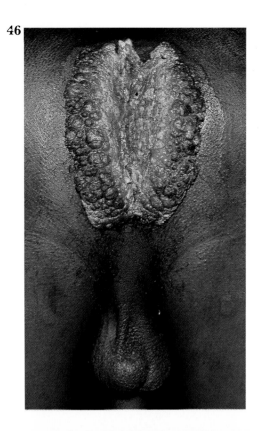

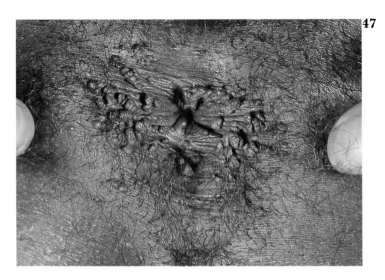

46 This young male prison inmate presented with venereal warts around the anus. He admitted rectal intercourse. Transmission of HIV in prisons is common.

47 This 18-year-old prisoner presented with multiple anal warts. He gave a history of frequent receptive anal intercourse while in the prison. He was HIV seropositive and had generalised lymphadenopathy.

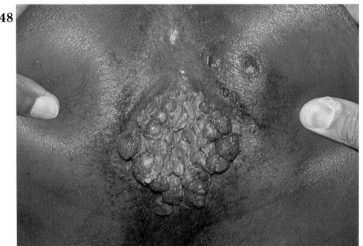

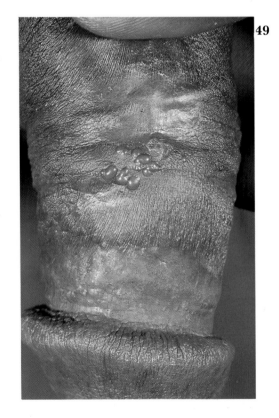

48 **Anal warts** in a bisexual man.

49 An example of "classical" herpes genitalis in a patient not infected with HIV.

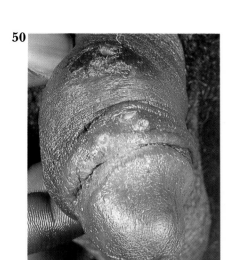

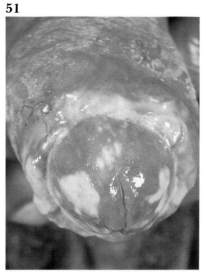

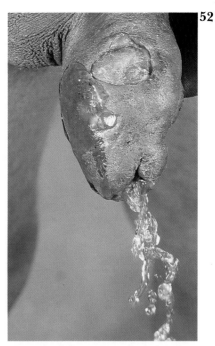

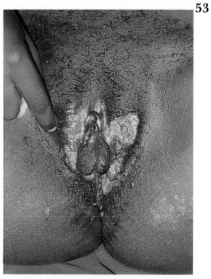

50 **Multiple superficial ulcers** after rupture of vesicles of herpes genitalis in a patient not infected with HIV.

51 Young male AIDS patient with pulmonary tuberculosis, weight loss and erosive non-healing ulcers of herpes on his genitalia.

52 This young man with ARC developed clusters of herpes lesions which became necrotic and led to a perforated prepuce. This illustration shows leakage of urine at the site of perforation.

53 **Erosive herpes genitalis** persisting for one month in a patient with AIDS.

54 & 55 **Chronic herpes genitalis** in a patient with AIDS.

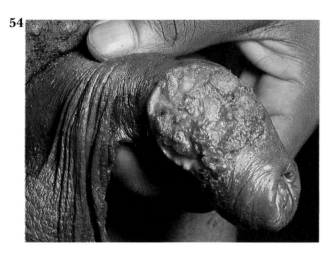

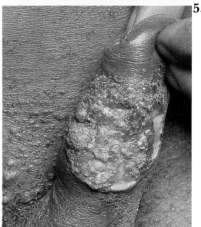

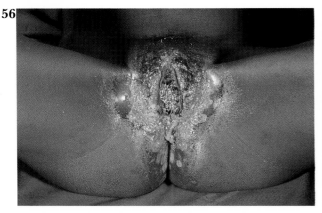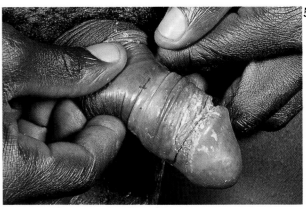

56 Erosive, extensive non-healing herpes genitalis in a patient with AIDS.

57 Recurrent candidal balanoposthitis in a patient with HIV disease. It responded temporarily to systemic ketoconazole therapy.

Section 8: Cutaneous Manifestations

Human immunodeficiency virus (HIV) infection, like most systemic infections, produces skin lesions which can often be used as cutaneous markers of disease. Recurrent bacterial, viral and fungal infections occur with increased frequency. Kaposi's sarcoma, multidermatomal and necrotic herpes zoster, drug reactions, extensive seborrhoeic dermatitis refractory to topical fluorinated corticosteroids and pruritic maculopapular eruptions are common manifestations of AIDS and ARC. Candidiasis, severe genital herpes,

extensive molluscum contagiosum and tinea are less frequent and usually refractory to treatment. In a study conducted in Lusaka, one or more cutaneous lesions occurred in 98% of the AIDS patients as compared to 53% of those with ARC. Multidermatomal herpes zoster and pruritic maculopapular eruption are highly associated with HIV-I infection in Zambia and Africa.

Differential diagnoses:

Herpes zoster

The unilateral painful eruption of grouped vesicles along a dermatome is typical. This distinctive clinical picture permits a diagnosis with little difficulty.

Seborrhoeic dermatitis

Manifests as dry flaky desquamation or as thick crusts on scalp, eyebrows, eyelids, nasolabial folds, lips, ears, sternal area, axillae and groin. Some cases may bear a close clinical resemblance to psoriasis, impetigo, generalised candidiasis and pityriasis rosea.

Psoriasis

Presents as symmetrical plaques covered with silvery white scales on the scalp, extensor surfaces of the limbs, elbows and knees. The nails are pitted.

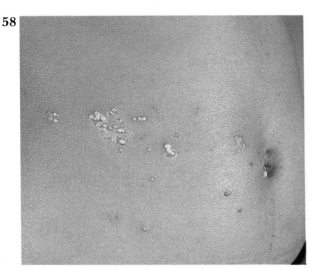

58 Scanty lesions of herpes zoster in a patient who was not infected with HIV.

Tinea corporis

The diagnosis is relatively easily made by finding fungi under the microscope in skin scrapings. Diseases which may resemble tinea corporis are pityriasis rosea, secondary syphilis, seborrhoeic dermatitis and psoriasis.

Molluscum contagiosum

This is characterised by central umbilication of the wartlike papular lesion.

Generalised candidiasis

Generally involves the genitocrural fold, anal region, axillae, hands and the feet. Seborrhoeic dermatitis and psoriasis may simulate cutaneous candidiasis.

Papular dermatoses of HIV

This rash generally occurs on the trunk in crops. It must be differentiated from papular urticaria from insect bites which occurs in crops usually on the arms and legs.

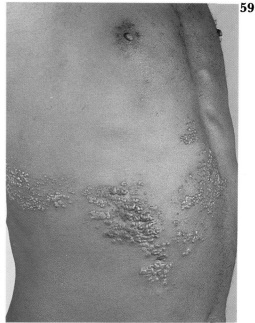

59

59 Multidermatomal herpes zoster in a HIV patient with generalised lymphadenopathy.

60 Multidermatomal herpes zoster in a patient who was receiving treatment for pulmonary tuberculosis.

61 This young man with AIDS presented with multidermatomal herpes zoster. Over the next 2 years he developed pulmonary tuberculosis and oral candidiasis.

60

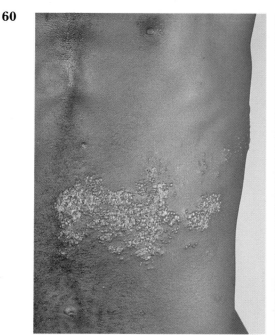

61

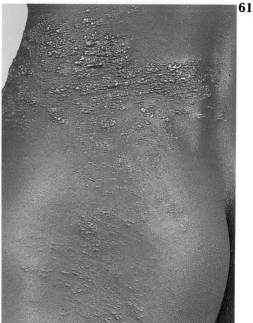

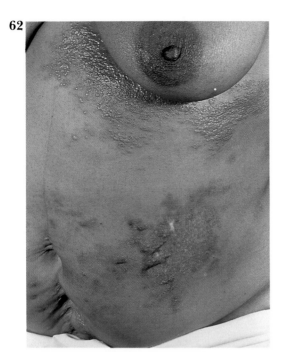

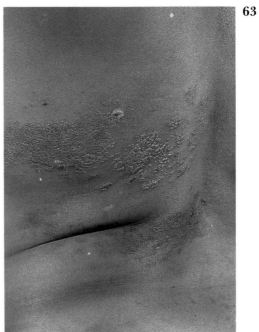

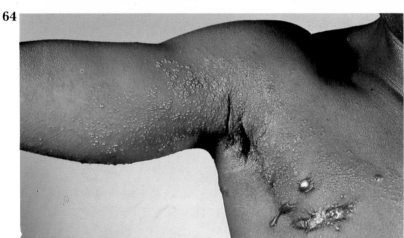

62 & 63 32-year-old female AIDS patient presented with multidermatomal herpes zoster. Six months later she presented with second episode of herpes zoster and persistent generalised lymphadenopathy. She died six months later.

64 & 65 Second episode of multidermatomal herpes zoster in a young patient.

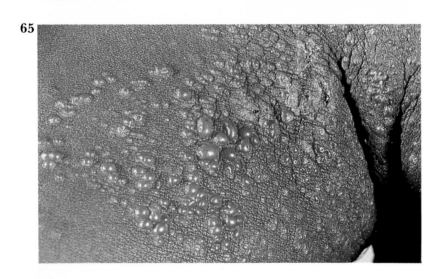

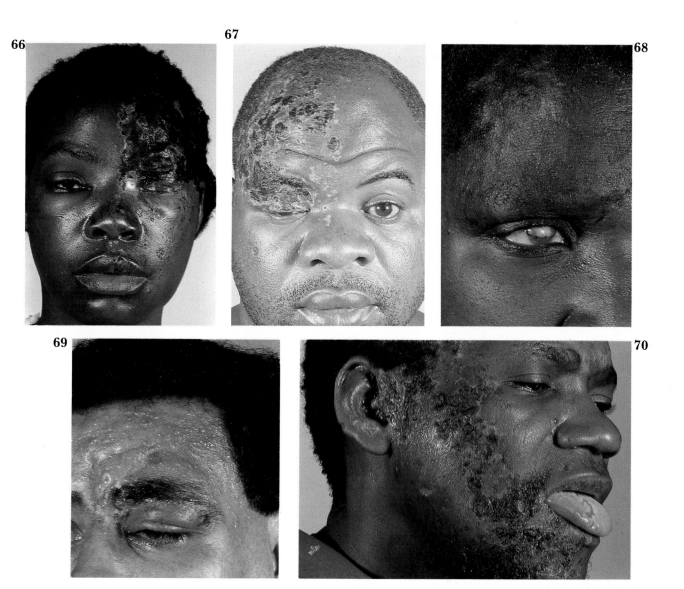

66 A patient with ophthalmic herpes zoster involving cornea of left eye, who rapidly progressed to AIDS.

67 **Ophthalmic herpes zoster** in a patient with ARC.

68 This patient with AIDS-related complex developed ophthalmic herpes zoster. The herpetic lesions healed with keratitis.

69 **Ophthalmic herpes zoster** in an Arab patient with ARC.

70 This young male AIDS patient who presented with herpes zoster and later developed keloid scars and generalised lymphadenopathy.

71 This 35-year-old AIDS patient developed ophthalmic herpes zoster which later disseminated. Subsequently, he developed a keloid and post-herpetic neuralgia.

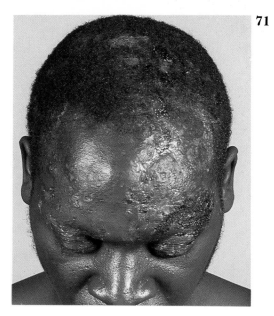

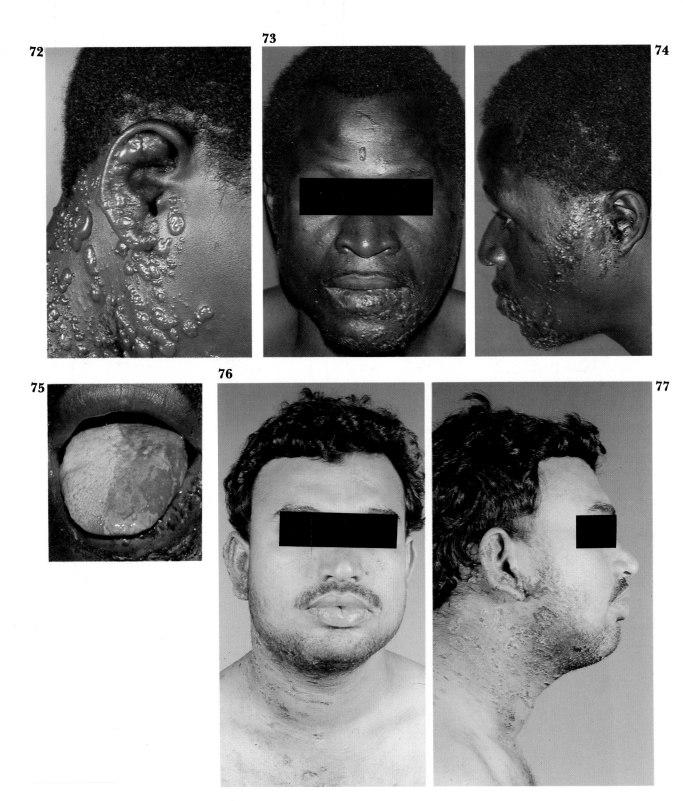

72 **Multidermatomal herpes** zoster with HIV infection.

73–75 **Herpes zoster** involving the facial nerve and tongue.

76 & 77 **Multidermatomal herpes zoster** in a young Asian patient.

78 Multidermatomal herpes zoster has a positive predictive value for HIV infection of almost 90%. The trunk is the usual site affected and herpetic neuralgia is common.

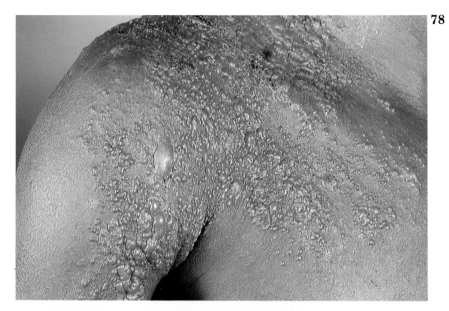

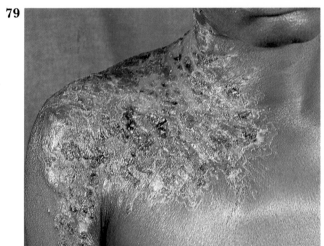

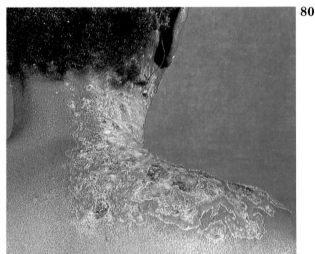

79 & 80 This 20-year-old man with AIDS presented with multidermatomal herpes zoster and buccal candidiasis. The lesions healed slowly over 4 weeks and was followed by extensive scarring and post-herpetic neuralgia.

81 Keloids from herpes zoster in an HIV patient.

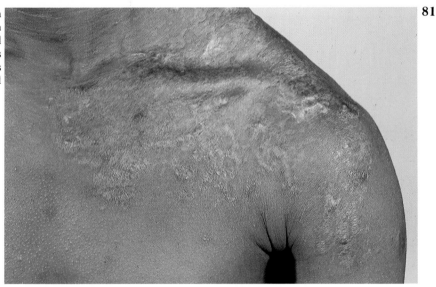

82

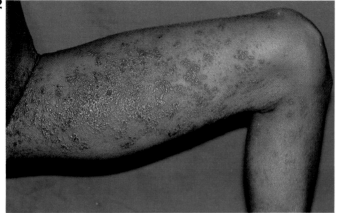

83

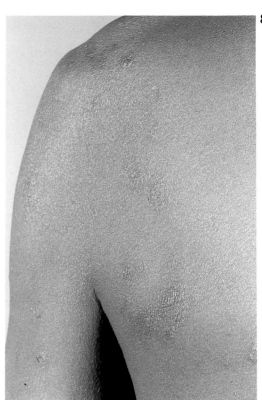

82 **Lesions of herpes zoster** on the third day after their onset in a young HIV infected woman.

83 **Drug eruptions** are common in patients with HIV disease. Here, a patient with AIDS-related complex developed eczematous eruption while being treated with co-trimoxazole.

84 & 85 **Cystic acne** in a patient with AIDS-related complex. Intralesional steroids are contraindicated.

86 **Fixed drug eruption** in a patient with HIV disease being treated with co-trimoxazole.

84

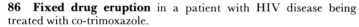

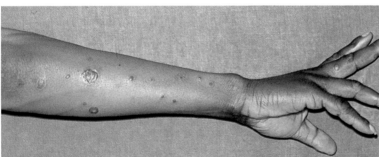

86

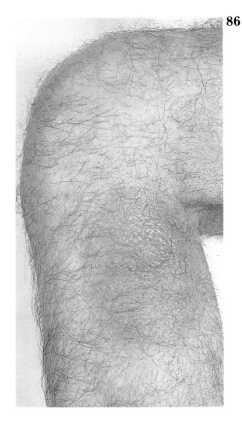

85

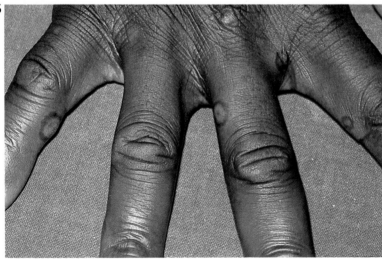

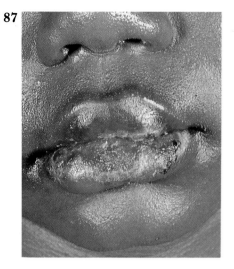

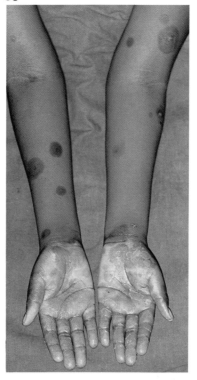

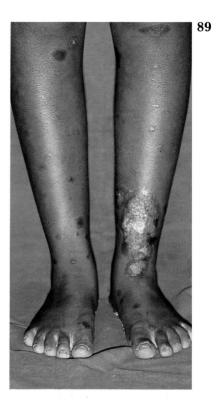

87–89 This patient with AIDS-related complex developed a fixed drug eruption while on tetracycline therapy.

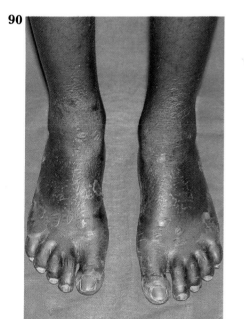

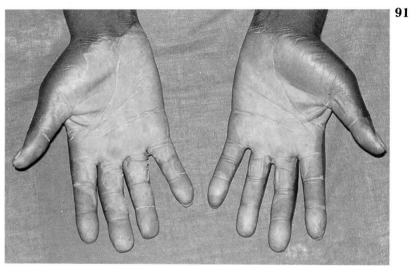

90 & 91 A patient with ARC who developed a fixed drug eruption while taking tetracycline.

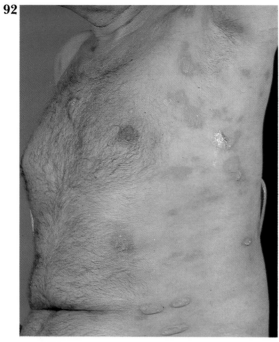

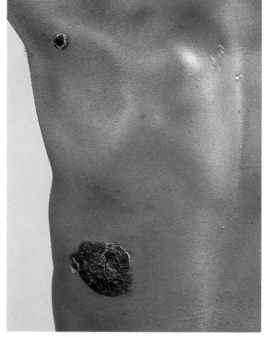

92 This middle-aged Asian man with ARC developed a fixed drug eruption while taking co-trimoxazole.

93 A fixed drug eruption due to co-trimoxazole.

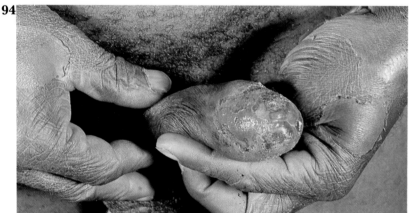

94 A fixed drug eruption due to co-trimoxazole in a patient with ARC. The hands and genitalia show annular lesions.

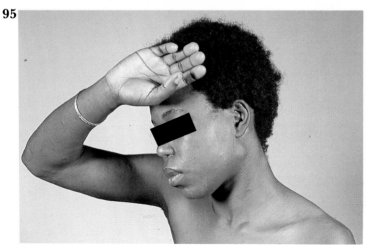

95 This patient had generalised lymphadenopathy and a drug reaction to co-trimoxazole.

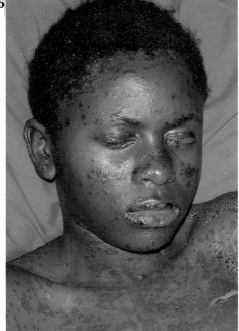

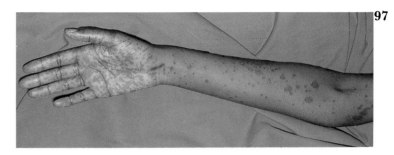

97 This 24-year-old HIV infected woman developed a drug eruption while being treated with co-trimoxazole for a chronic cough. The eruption cleared on discontinuation of the co-trimoxazole and after a short course of systemic steroid therapy.

96 This young woman developed Stevens-Johnson syndrome while receiving treatment for pulmonary tuberculosis. The likely offending drugs were streptomycin and thiacetazone. Management includes discontinuation of all drugs and after Stevens-Johnson syndrome has cleared, reintroduction of alternative drugs for treatment of tuberculosis.

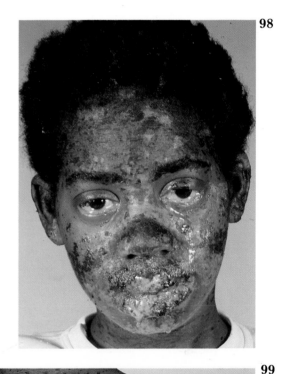

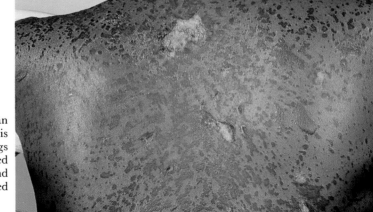

98 & 99 This young HIV infected woman on therapy for pulmonary tuberculosis developed a drug eruption. Although drugs were promptly discontinued, she developed inflammation of conjunctiva, nasal and buccal mucosae. Her condition improved following systemic steroids.

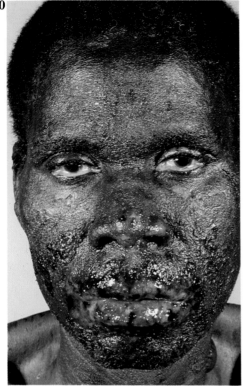

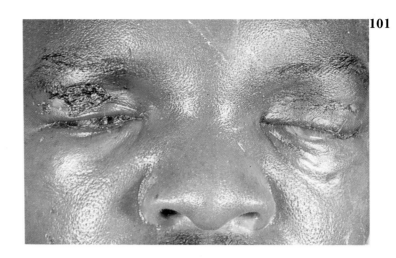

100 An AIDS patient with Stevens-Johnson syndrome who was on treatment for pulmonary tuberculosis. Systemic steroids are contraindicated.

101 Stevens-Johnson syndrome man with AIDS. He was receiving streptomycin, isoniazid, thiacetazone and rifampicin for pulmonary tuberculosis.

102 & 103 Seborrhoeic dermatitis in patients with ARC.

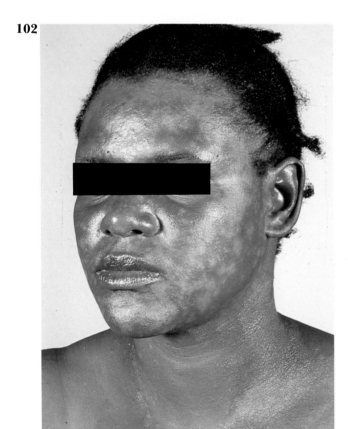

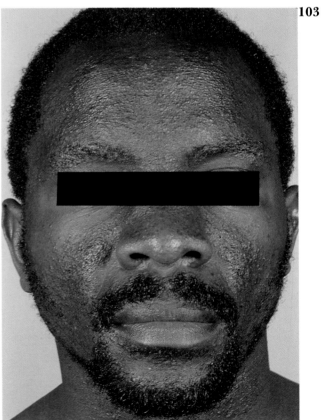

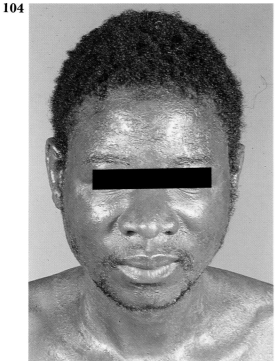

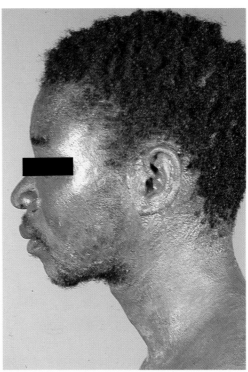

104 & 105 This young man presented with disseminated seborrhoeic dermatitis. Since it is an HIV-related dermatosis, it did not respond to conventional topical steroids.

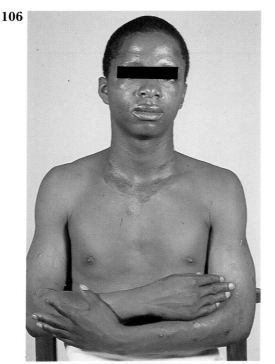

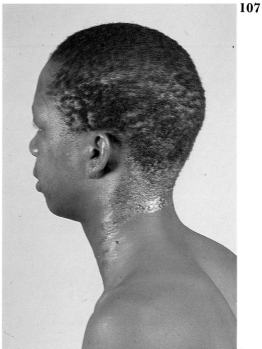

106 & 107 **Weeping lesions of acute seborrhoeic dermatitis** in which there is evidence of a photosensitive element. When seborrhoeic dermatitis presents in association with HIV disease, the condition is often unresponsive to treatment with topical steroids. Systemic steroids are contra-indicated.

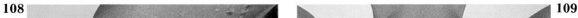

108
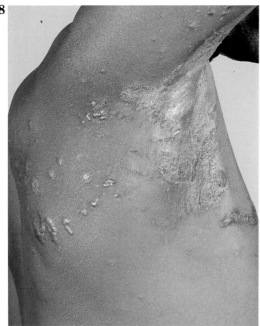

109
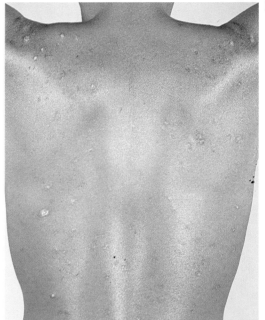

110
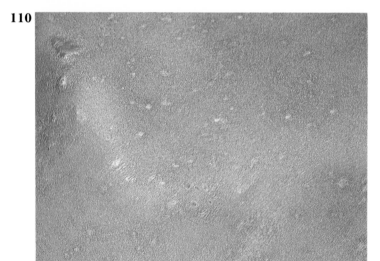

111
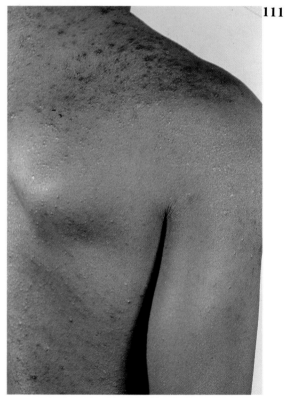

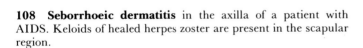

108 Seborrhoeic dermatitis in the axilla of a patient with AIDS. Keloids of healed herpes zoster are present in the scapular region.

109 This 35-year-old man with ARC presented with fever, chronic cough and itchy maculo-papular dermatosis. Fresh crops of lesions continued to appear for 8-10 weeks.

110 A maculo-papular eruption in a patient with AIDS showing atrophic scars.

111 This man with ARC had a history of chronic cough, generalised lymphadenopathy and an itchy maculo-papular dermatosis.

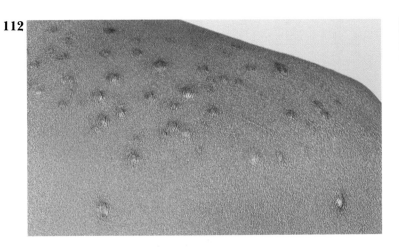

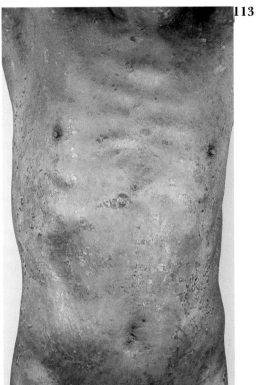

112 A young man with ARC who developed crops of itchy papular lesions. Fresh crops continued to appear for 3 months.

113–115 This 35-year-old patient with AIDS had history of chronic diarrhoea and weight loss and developed a bullous dermatosis which responded to dapsone therapy.

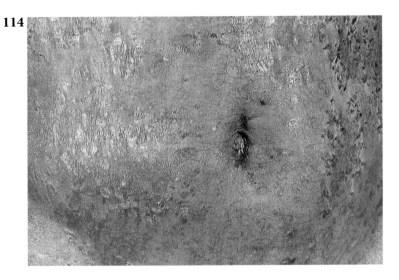

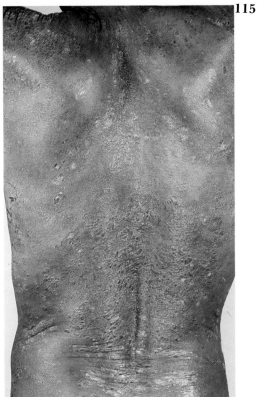

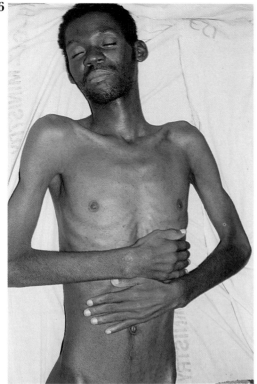

116 Weight loss, papular dermatosis and pigmentation of the sun-exposed areas in a patient with AIDS.

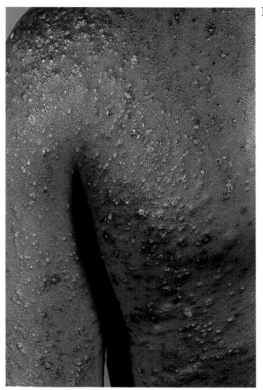

117 Multiple papular lesions on the back of a patient with ARC.

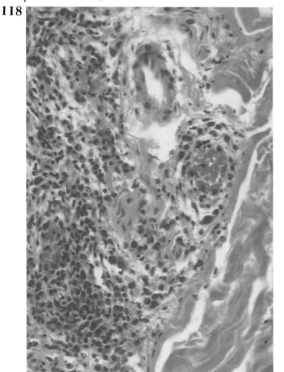

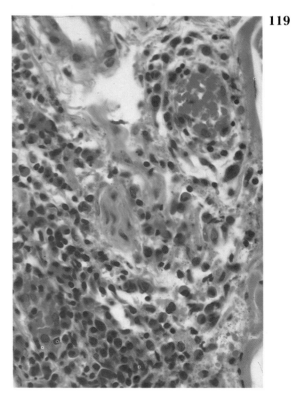

118 & 119 Histology of maculo-papular dermatosis showing a lympho-plasmacytic angiitis (by courtesy of Dr. A. Macher, Armed Forces Institute of Pathology, Bethesda, USA).

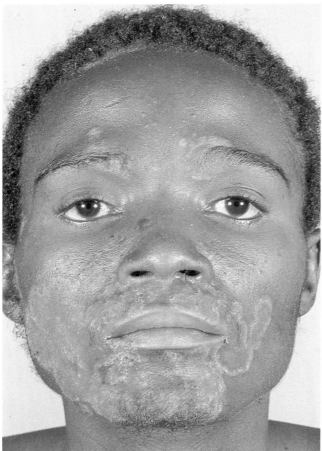

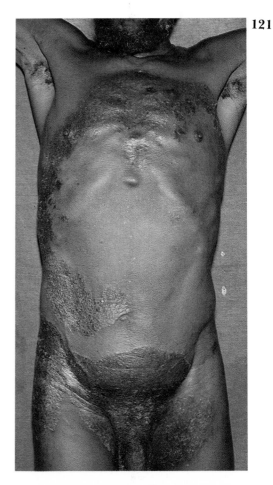

120 Annular lesions of tinea imbricata in a patient with ARC. The lesions were healed by oral ketoconazole therapy.

121 This young patient with AIDS had multiple pigmented pruritic lesions of dermatophyte infection.

122 Extensive dermatophyte infection in an 18-year-old woman with ARC.

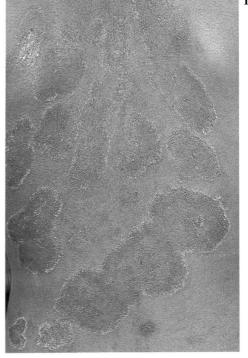

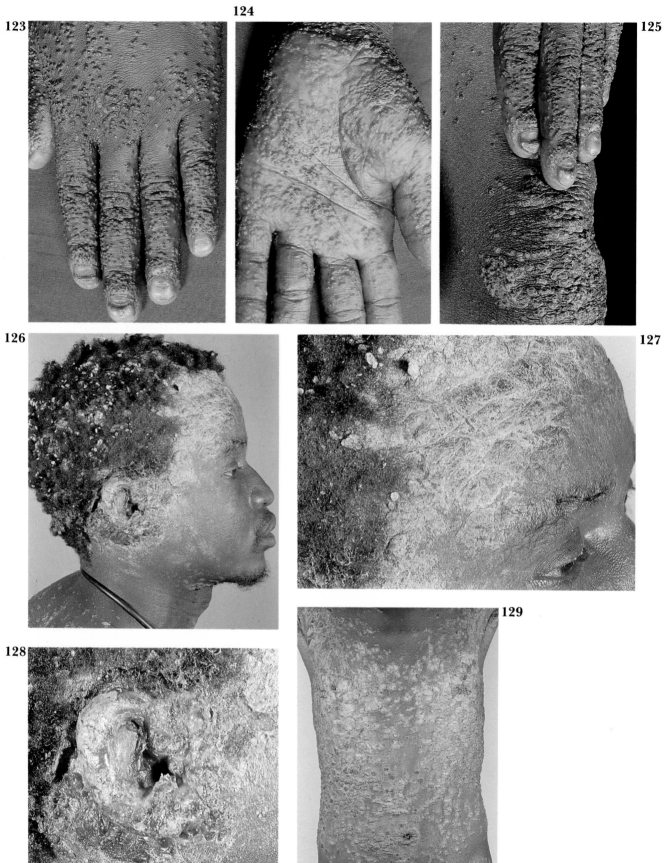

130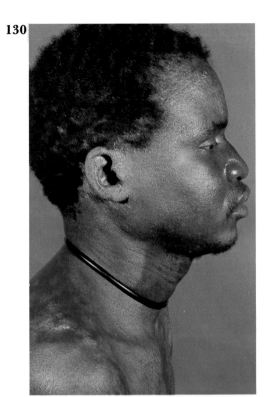

131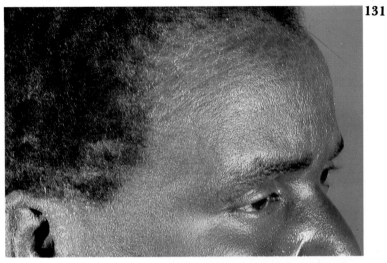

133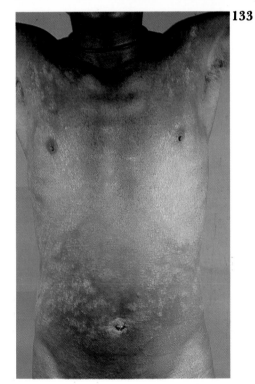

132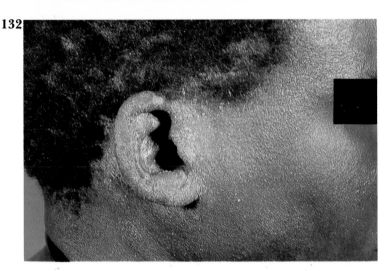

123–125 This 20-year-old woman with ARC developed an id eruption from a dermatophyte infection on her trunk and toe webs.

126–129 A 28-year-old male patient with ARC who presented with generalised lymphadenopathy, recurrent diarrhoea and extensive scaly plaques of psoriasis.

130–133 The same patient after treatment with antibiotics and topical steroids.

45

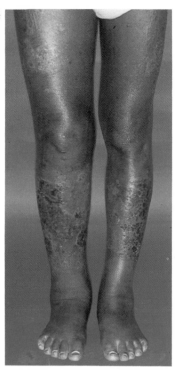 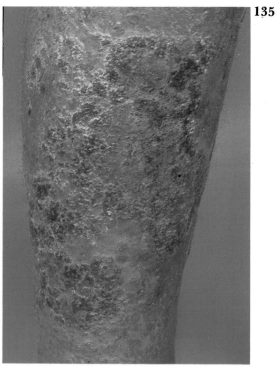
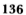

134 **Psoriasis** worsens in some patients with HIV infection. This patient has AAKS as well, which is responsible for the oedema of his right leg.

135 Close up view of 134.

136–138 This 30-year-old man with ARC presented with extensive psoriatic lesions on his scalp, face, trunk and extremities. He also had generalised lymphadenopathy and a history of chronic fever.

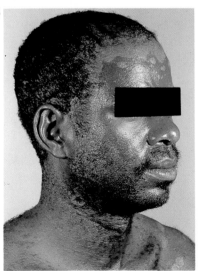 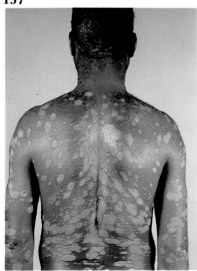 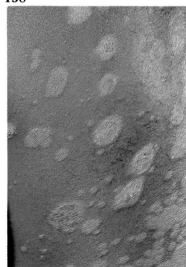

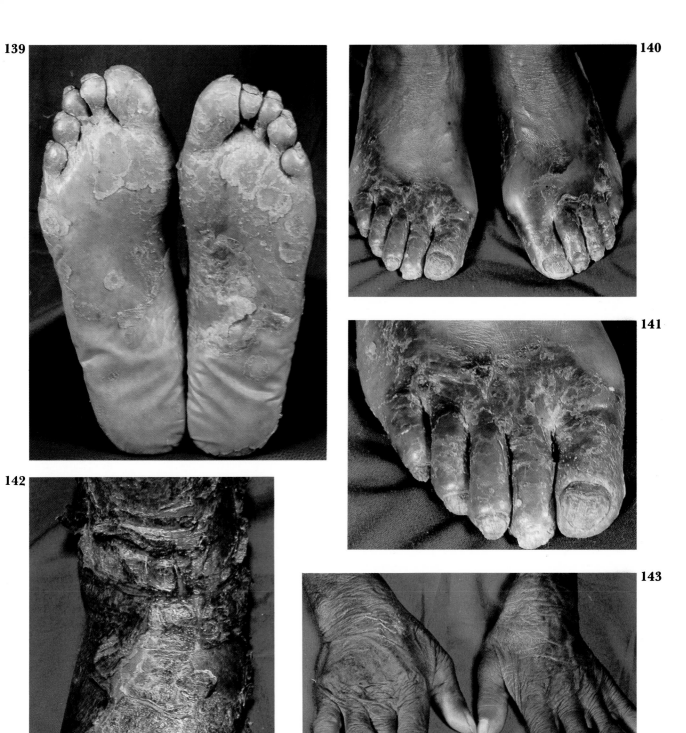

139–141 Cutaneous candidiasis in a patient with AIDS. Response to ketoconazole therapy was good.

142 & 143 A malnourished AIDS patient with chronic diarrhoea who developed severe pellagra dermatitis.

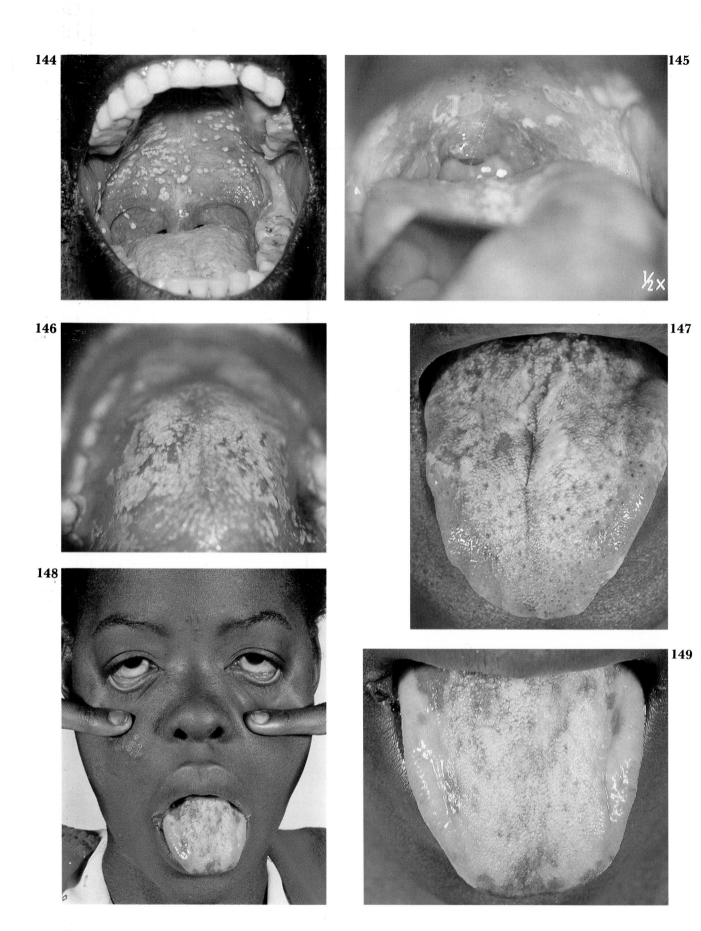

144 Extensive oral candidiasis in a patient who had pulmonary tuberculosis, weight loss and chronic diarrhoea.

145 A young woman with AIDS who had a history of recurrent diarrhoea, fever, and weight loss, developed erythematous, flaky spots on her palate and buccal mucosa. She also had generalised lymphadenopathy.

146 This young man with AIDS had a history of chronic diarrhoea, weight loss and recurrent fever and presented with 'curdy' flakes on his hard palate.

147 A patient with ARC who had a black hairy tongue caused by papilloma virus. The patient was unaware of these lesions.

148 This young woman with AIDS had a tuberculous pleural effusion and pigmented, filiform plaques on her tongue, tinea corporis on her right cheek and herpes labialis on the right angle of her mouth. She also had pigmentation of her conjunctivae.

149 Close-up of the tongue of the patient in **148**.

150 This young man with HIV-disease has pigmented, filiform lesions on his tongue.

151 & 152 A 21-year-old woman who presented with venereal warts and generalised lymphadenopathy. She complained of weight loss and diarrhoea. The illustrations show hairy leucoplakia on her tongue which is caused by Epstein-Barr virus.

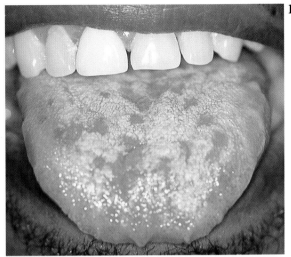

150

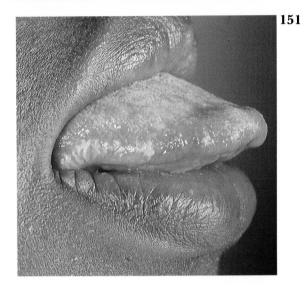

151

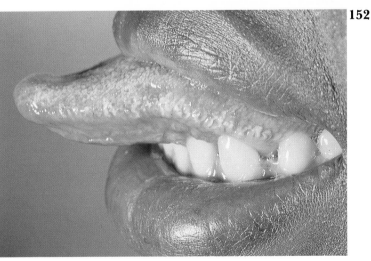

152

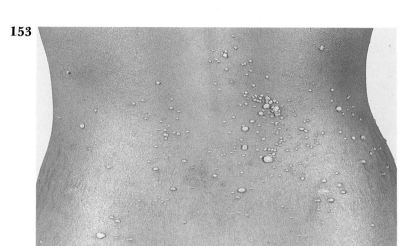

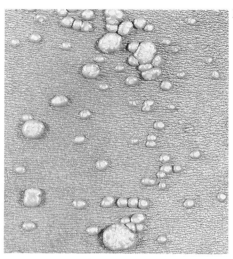

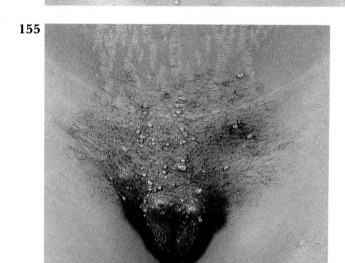

153–155 This 20-year-old woman with AIDS presented with history of recurrent diarrhoea, chronic cough and weight loss. Physical examination revealed generalised umbilicated papules of molluscum contagiosum.

156 Multiple umbilicated papules of molluscum contagiosum on the face of a young adult patient, who later developed AAKS.

157 Multiple umbilicated papules of molluscum contagiosum on the popliteal fossae. The lesions can be missed if careful dermatological examination is not done. Non-genital molluscum in an adult is suggestive of moderate to severe immune suppression.

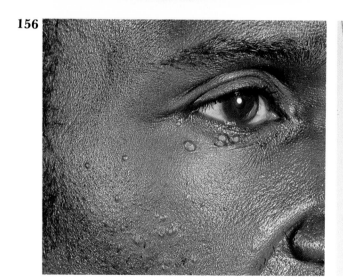

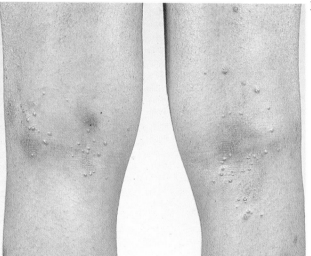

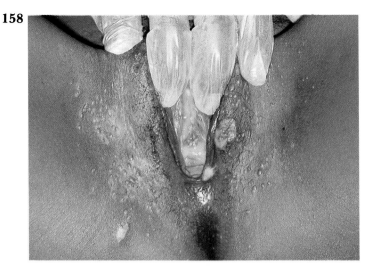

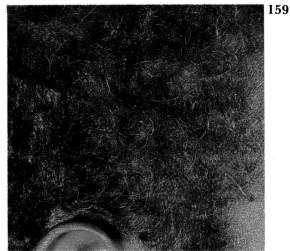

159

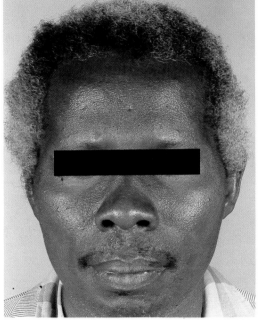

160

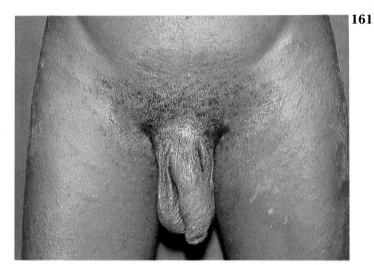

161

162

158 Young patient with AIDS who had concomitant herpes genitalis and umbilicated papules of molluscum contagiosum which subsequently disseminated to involve trunk and face.

159 Young patient with AIDS who had sparse, brittle and lustreless hair on the scalp.

160 39-year-old man had grey hair when first seen which is most unusual in a Zambian of his age. During his response to chemotherapy for AAKS, the normal black pigmentation reappeared at the roots of his hair.

161 & 162 This young man with HIV-related disease had recalcitrant seborrhoeic dermatitis involving scalp, face and pubic region. He had candidal intertrigo in the groin and yellow discolouration of the distal nails.

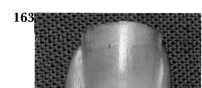

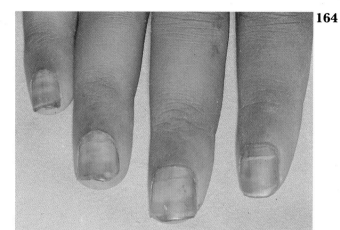

163 A patient with tuberculous pleural effusion showing yellow nails with lymphoedema of the nail fold.

164 Violet or yellow nail discolouration seen as a band along distal portion of nail plate in a patient with AIDS. There was no associated lung pathology. This manifestation is probably due to vasculitis of the nail bed.

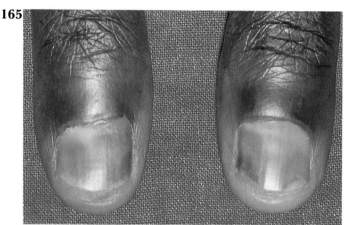

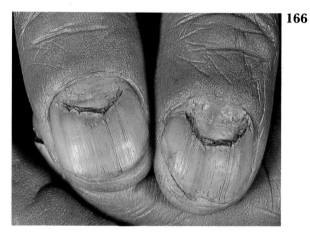

165 A young girl with pulmonary tuberculosis and HIV-related disease developed yellow discolouration of the distal parts of her nail plates. This was associated with onycholysis of nail plate and lymphoedema of nail folds.

166 This young man with ARC developed psoriasis and deep pitting of his nails.

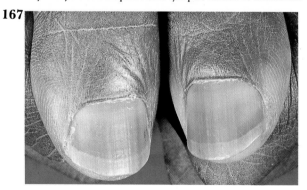

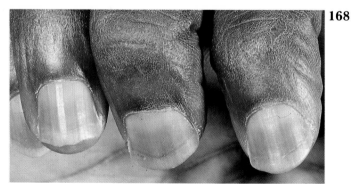

167 & 168 Yellow nail changes in a patient with chronic diarrhoea.

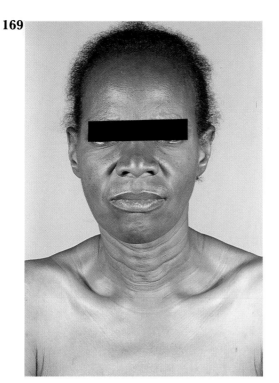

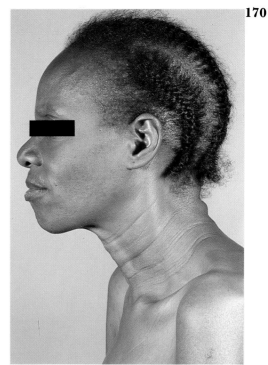

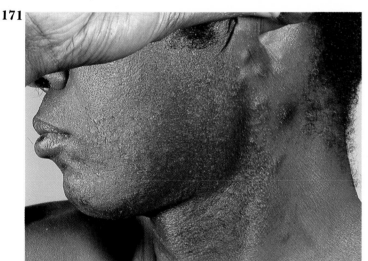

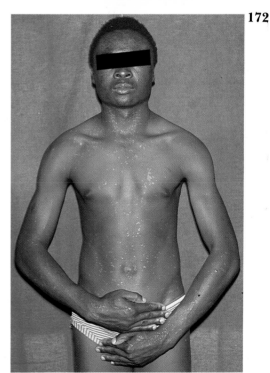

169 & 170 In patients with AIDS, weight loss, hair changes and diffuse pigmentation of the face are commonly seen.

171 This patient has cutaneous nodules of AAKS behind and below his ear, and darkening of the skin of his face and neck. This has been seen in only a few patients with AAKS and its significance is unknown.

172 A patient with AIDS-related complex who developed extensive flat topped papules diagnosed as plane warts.

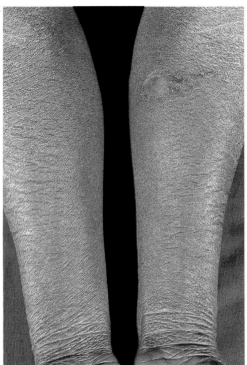

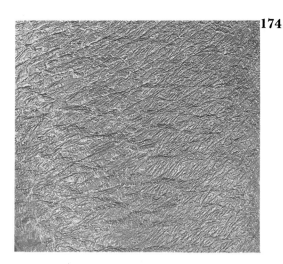

173 & 174 This young man with ARC, who had had flexural eczema for 2 years, developed erythroderma while on treatment for his eczema.

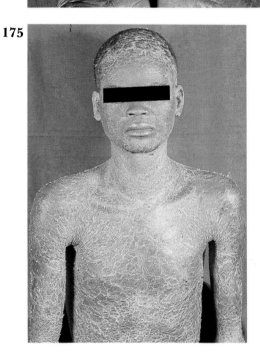

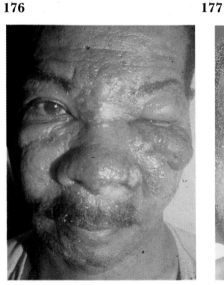

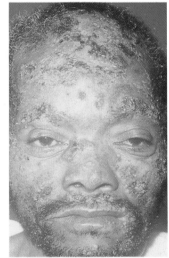

175 This 20-year-old HIV-infected man presented with psoriatic erythroderma of acute onset. He later developed arthropathy.

176 & 177 Disseminated American cutaneous leishmaniasis in Brazilian men with AIDS, seen as multiple erythematous, non-ulcerative nodules on the face. The species was identified as L. braziliensis. (By courtesy of Dr. J. Rodrigues Coura, Instituto Oswaldo Cruz, Rio de Janeiro, Brazil).

Section 9: AIDS-related Complex (ARC)

HIV disease is a continuum. The AIDS-related complex includes symptoms and signs occurring in a person with an HIV infection which reflects the progressive breakdown of immune competence, with or without evidence of infection of the central nervous system.

The common features of ARC are symmetrical lymph node enlargement, mild weight loss, recurrent diarrhoea, malaise and fatigue, drenching night sweats, repeated episodes of oral candidiasis, herpes zoster, fungal skin eruptions, and repeated episodes of infection which usually bring the patient to either a physician or a surgeon. Examination of the mouth shows one or more abnormalities in the majority of patients and oral hairy leukoplakia caused by Epstein-Barr virus is pathognomonic of HIV infection.

Individual bacterial and fungal infections usually respond slowly to standard treatment and they tend to recur. These illnesses interfere with work and enjoyment, but do not threaten life.

Symptoms of neurologic involvement are uncommon but careful physical examination may detect abnormal signs with a paradoxical pattern.

Laboratory investigations show lymphopoenia in adults (but not children) with a progressive reduction in absolute numbers of T4 lymphocytes. Mild anaemia (haemoglobin 8-11 gm/dl) is common. Thrombocytopoenia is observed in a few patients and transfusions may be required to control haemorrhage.

Differential diagnoses:

Leucoplakia of debilitation

This whitish discolouration of the mucous membrane of the mouth is associated with malnutrition due to chronic ill health.

Leucopoenia

Leucocytosis is often a sign of bacterial infection but in overwhelming infections, leucopoenia may be present.

Drug-induced leucopoenia

Patients with AIDS may have drug induced leucopoenia resulting from treatment of opportunistic infections. However leucopoenia with AIDS occurs in the absence of drugs.

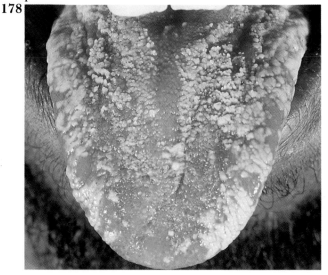

178 A patient with pulmonary tuberculosis, weight loss, generalised lymphadenopathy and extensive oral candidiasis.

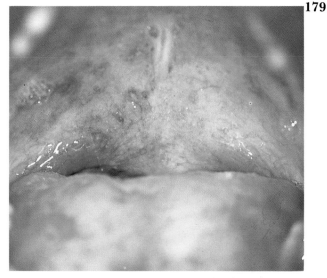

179 This woman presented with weight loss and persistent generalised lymphadenopathy. She had erythema of the anterior pillars of the fauces, and erythematous patches on the palate probably due to candidiasis.

180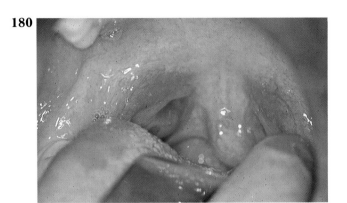

181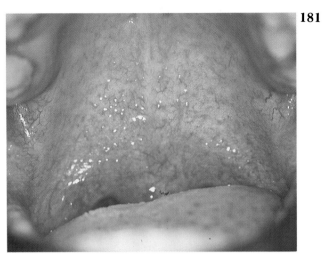

180 This patient had atypical Kaposi's sarcoma of the lymph nodes. No tumour is visible in the intra-oral photograph which shows erythema of the anterior pillars of the fauces. This is seen often in HIV-infected patients.

182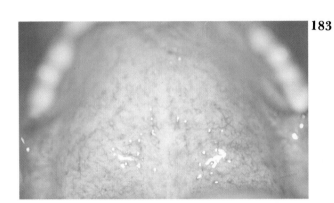

183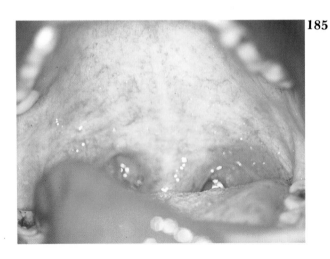

181–183 Patchy erythema of the mucosa of the hard palate is common in HIV patients. The nature of the pathology is unknown.

184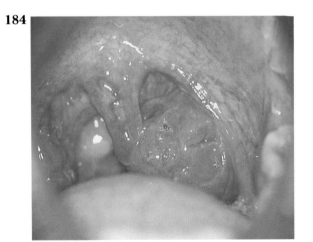

185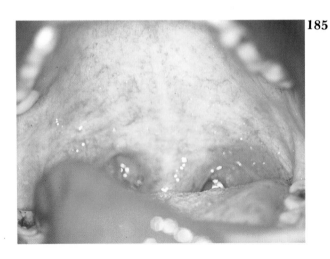

184 Marked hypertrophy of the tonsils occurs in some HIV positive patients in association with persistent generalised lymphadenopathy, but it is often more symmetrical than it is in this picture.

185 Patients with persistent generalised lymphadenopathy may have hyperaemia of the anterior pillars of the fauces, and prominent vascular markings on the palate.

186 This AIDS patient presented with black hairy tongue, herpes simplex, tinea corporis, generalised lymphadenopathy and genital molluscum contagiosum. This illustration shows the oral candidiasis.

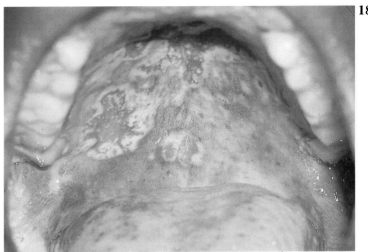

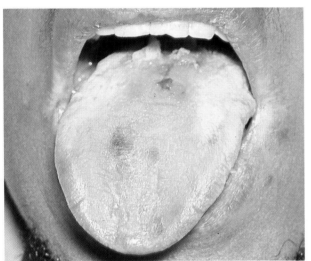

187 The tongue is dry and shrunken because of dehydration, and coated with candida: a common combination.

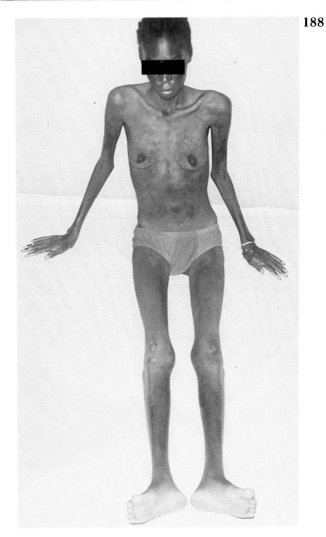

188 This young woman with AIDS presented with lesions of porphyria cutanea tarda. She had gross weight loss and arthropathy of both knees.

Section 10: Kaposi's Sarcoma

Endemic Kaposi's Sarcoma (KS) in Africa has a wide variety of manifestations, ranging from a few nodules on a slightly swollen foot to destructive infiltration of whole limbs, but the natural history and response to treatment are predictable, and the diagnosis is easy to make.

Against this background a change in the pattern of presentation and behaviour of Kaposi's sarcoma has occurred since 1983, reported first in Zambia, but observed later in Uganda, Zimbabwe and Malawi. Patients with endemic KS continue to present as in the past, but in addition growing numbers of patients have been seen with unusual symptoms and signs, and rapidly progressive disease. This pattern of presentation will be referred to as atypical African Kaposi's sarcoma (AAKS).

Patients with AAKS are younger (mean age 27 years) than those with KS (mean 41 years); they are more likely to be female (sex ratio M:F 3:1 compared with more than 10:1 for endemic KS), and histories are of shorter duration, (mean 9 months compared to 31 months). At least half of patients with AAKS have no peripheral nodules whatsoever, and those with skin lesions have plaques on the trunk, face, genitalia or proximal parts of limbs, all unusual sites for disease in KS.

The commonest presenting symptom in AAKS is generalised symmetrical lymph node enlargement. Two thirds of patients have one or more opportunistic infections (usually oral candidiasis or genital ulceration) at diagnosis. Weight loss is common, and so are plaques of Kaposi's sarcoma in the mouth, particularly on the hard palate.

Pleural effusions are detectable in about 25% of patients and others develop respiratory distress associated with infiltration of the perihilar and lower zones on chest radiographs.

A few patients have conjunctival KS nodules, hepatic or splenic enlargement, swollen tonsils, a pericardial effusion or encephalopathy which is probably due to the primary HIV infection, not secondary opportunists. The most striking difference between AAKS and KS is the aggressive behaviour of the new disease: an initial response to chemotherapy with Actinomycin D and Vincristine is seen in 60% of patients but often ceases after a few weeks. There is a high early mortality (median survival 7.5 months) in patients with poor prognostic signs which are weight loss in excess of 10kg, oedema of head or trunk, pulmonary infiltration or encephalopathy.

Differential diagnoses:

Mycosis fungoides

This is a rare T-cell lymphoma which invades the skin. It appears as a brown itchy, scaly or nodular lesion. Biopsy of the lesion will distinguish it from KS.

Generalised lymphadenopathy of disseminated tuberculosis

There are many causes of generalised lymphadenopathy in the tropics. Infection such as tuberculosis and neoplastic diseases must be excluded.

Lymphoedema of feet due to other causes e.g. deep vein thrombosis

Careful examination will distinguish this from other causes.

189–192 Lymph node enlargement in Kaposi's sarcoma is symmetrical around the sagittal plane, as in this patient, but individual nodes are rarely as large as shown here. The patient's general health is undisturbed and he has not lost weight.

Aged 20 when first seen in August 1981 with massive symmetrical lymphadenopathy and scanty peripheral skin lesions, this presentation was interpreted as the "childhood" lymphadenopathic variant of endemic Kaposi's sarcoma occurring at an unusual age. Chemotherapy was given and an objective response followed. The patient returned in 1987, wasted and severely ill with recurrent lymphadenopathic disease. On this occasion his blood was positive for antibody to HIV. Serum from 1981 was not available for testing. In retrospect this patient is probably the first in Lusaka with Atypical African Kaposi's Sarcoma.

189

190

191

192

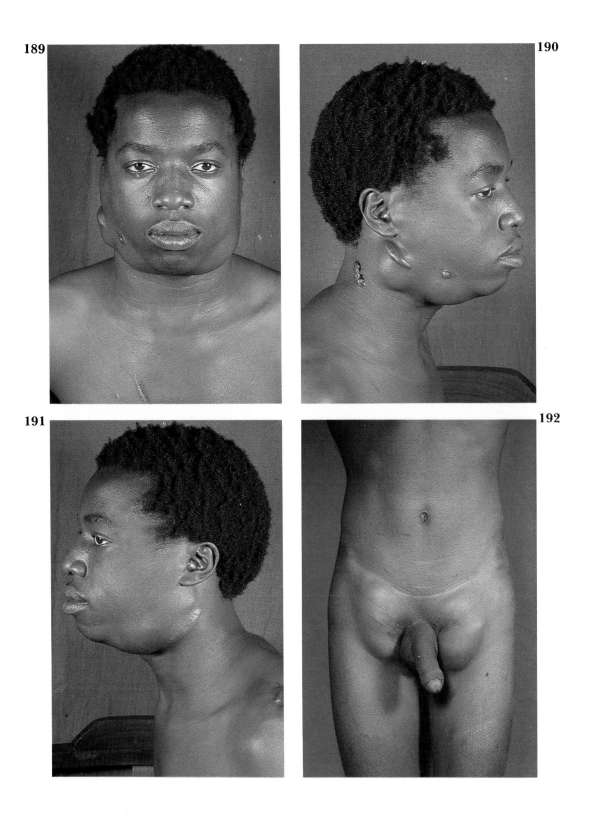

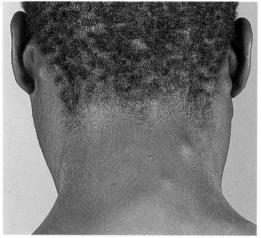

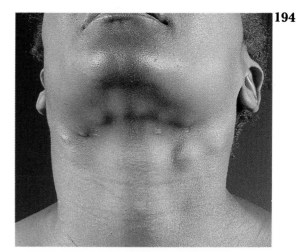

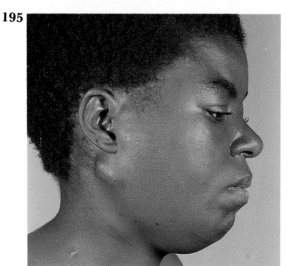

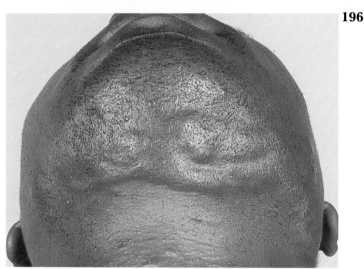

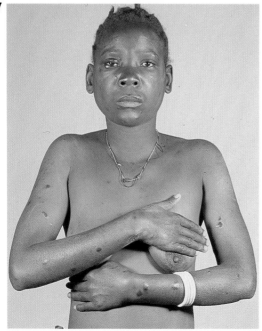

193 **Occipital lymph nodes** are often enlarged in AAKS, but usually more symmetrically than in this photograph.

194 **Symmetrical lymphadenopathy** in a woman patient with Kaposi's sarcoma seen in September 1982. Atypical disease was recognised as a distinct entity in 1983.

195 **Lymph nodes** enlarged by AAKS.

196 **Submandibular lymphadenopathy** in AAKS.

197 **Plaques** on both arms and face.

198 **Plaques** are particularly common in clusters around the ears, sometimes accompanied by darkening of the facial skin. Plaques are usually less dense on the trunk and neck.

199–206 Patient of mixed parentage with a lightly pigmented skin showing the purple colour of plaques, which are similar to those seen in Caucasian patients. He had no treatment over a six month period: note slow weight loss and the persistence of plaques on the trunk although they show an unusual loss of colour centrally.

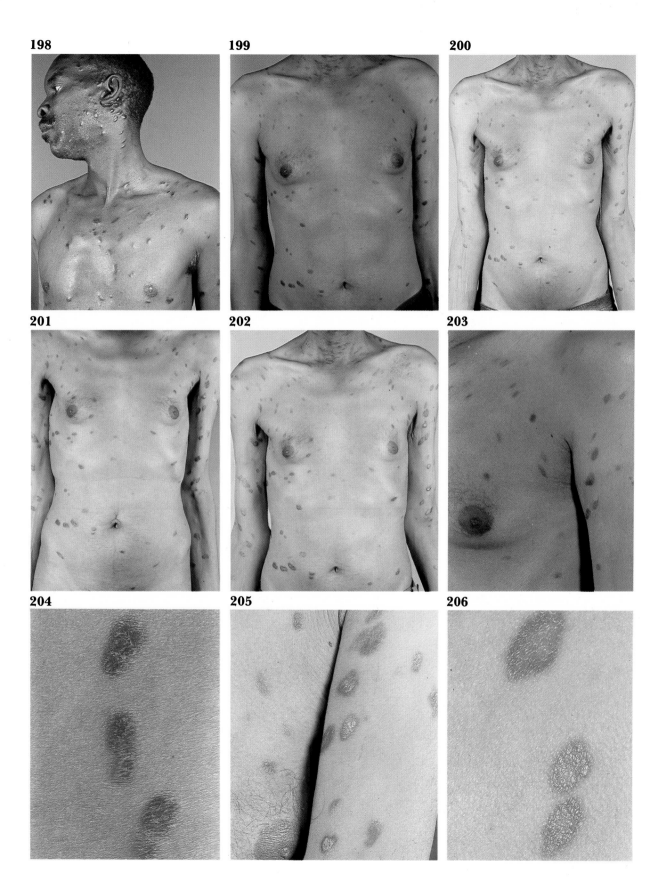

198

199

200

201

202

203

204

205

206

61

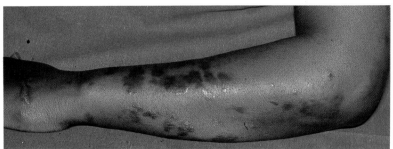

207 Irregularly shaped, darkly pigmented plaques are the commonest skin lesion of AAKS.

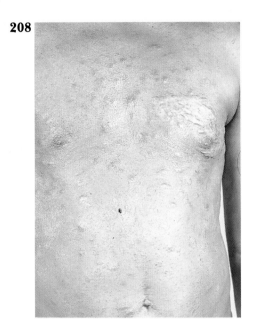

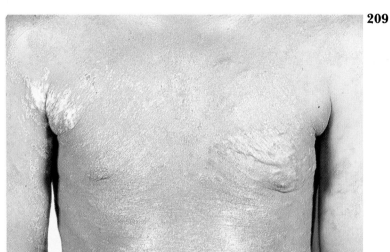

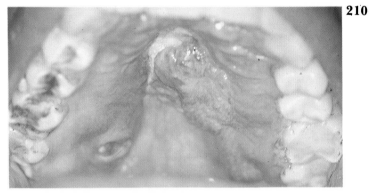

208–212 A 35-year-old man with psoriasis was on immuno-suppressive therapy since 1980 He developed herpes zoster in 1985 and complained of genital ulcers. Examination revealed vascular nodules on glans penis, and multiple vascular plaques on the palate.

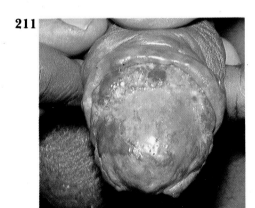

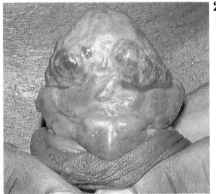

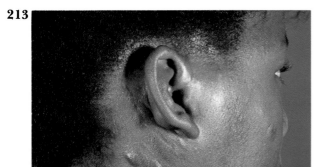

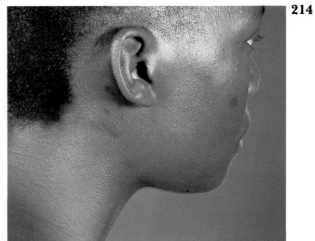

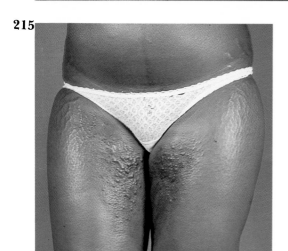

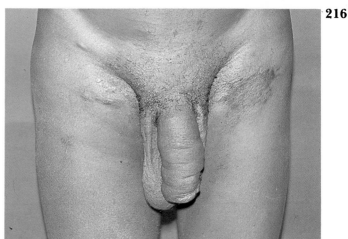

213–215 Two photographs taken eight weeks apart show regression of facial plaques following chemotherapy for AAKS. However, infiltration in both thighs and oral candidiasis persisted, and this woman's disease progressed, ending fatally three months later.

216 **Plaques on the thighs** and groin are often accompanied by oedema of the genitalia.

217 **Atypical African Kaposi's Sarcoma:** An early patient showing plaques in previously rare sites: the medial aspects of both thighs and both groins. Note that although both legs are severely oedematous, with peau d'orange, the genitalia are not.

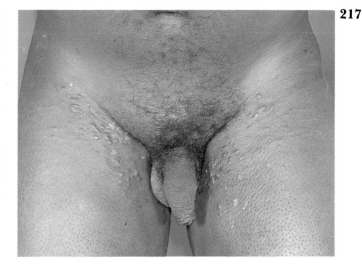

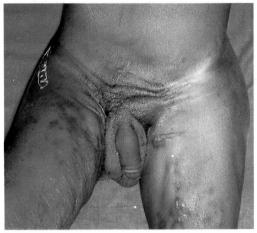

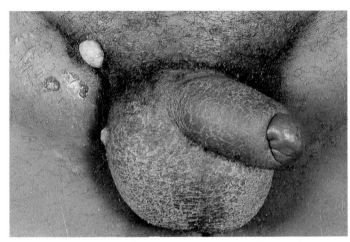

218 Plaques on medial aspects of both thighs, which are oedematous, with infiltration in both groins but no oedema of the external genitalia.

219 AAKS in a patient with AIDS. He had generalised lymphadenopathy, oedema of penis and scrotum, and vascular nodules in the groin.

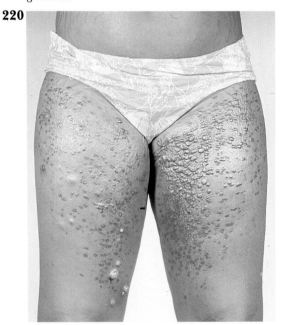

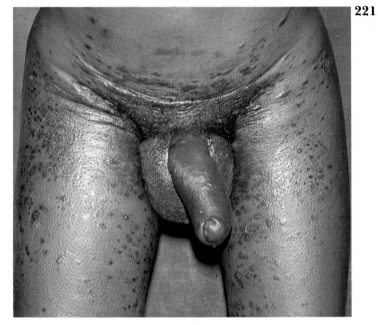

220 This 23-year-old woman had multiple vascular nodules of AAKS on her thighs. She also had generalised lymphadenopathy. Her HIV serology test was positive.

221 This 26-year-old man presented with swelling of both thighs and a 'saxophone' penis. Examination revealed 'woody' oedema of vascular nodules on the thighs. He had generalized lymphadenopathy and his HIV serologic test was positive.

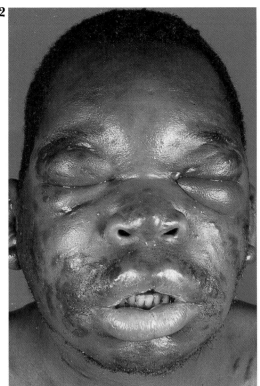

222

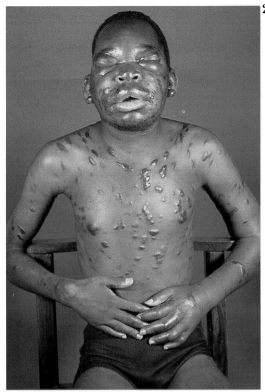

223

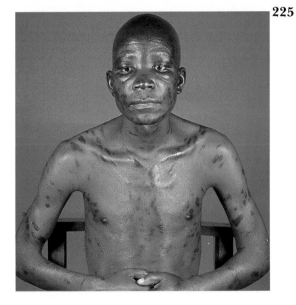

224

225

222–225 This young man was admitted with gross swelling of his head, neck and severe respiratory distress with parenchymal lung infiltration on chest radiographs. Plaques, facial oedema and respiratory distress responded to treatment with Actinomycin D and Vincristine initially, but symptoms and signs recurred about four months after the start of treatment and he died less than six months from diagnosis.

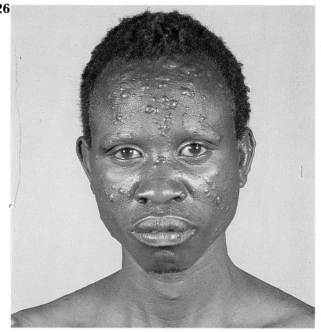

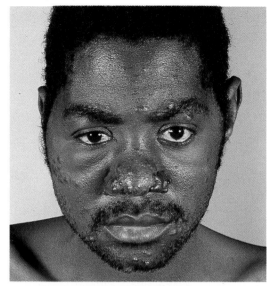

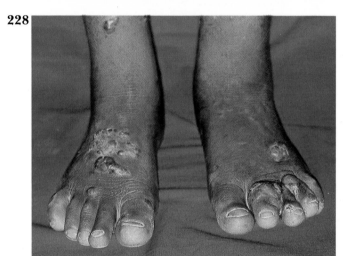

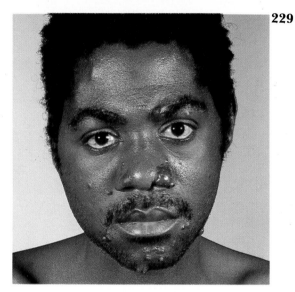

226 Although plaques are the commonest lesions of facial AAKS, nodules do occur, but very rarely ulcerate; note their nearly symmetrical distribution.

227 & 228 **KS lesions** on this man's face are more nodular than is usual. There are also a few plaques on his feet.

229 & 230 Same patient as in 227 seven months later with irregular, ulcerated plaques at typical sites on the hard palate.

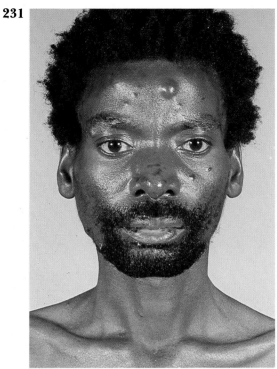

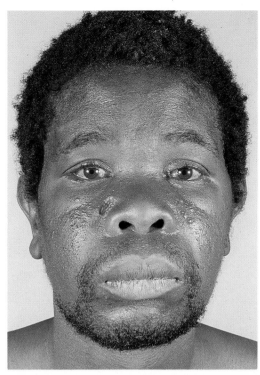

231 Note wasting, and facial nodules in addition to the more usual KS plaques on the tip of this man's nose.

232–234 This 34-year-old man has lesions of atypical Kaposi's Sarcoma on the face, with subconjunctival haemorrhages that are sometimes seen in association with thrombocytopoenia. His upper gums are replaced by masses of Kaposi's Sarcoma tissue.

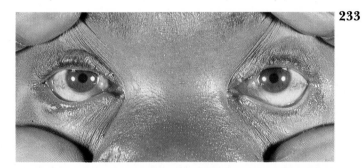

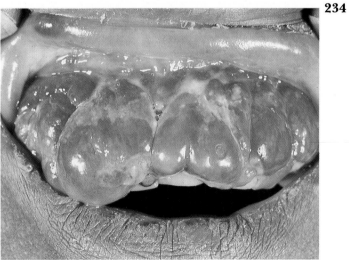

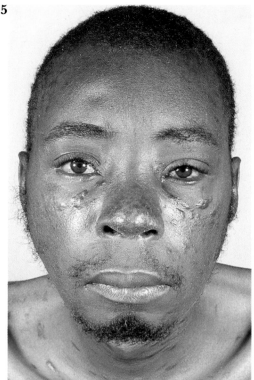

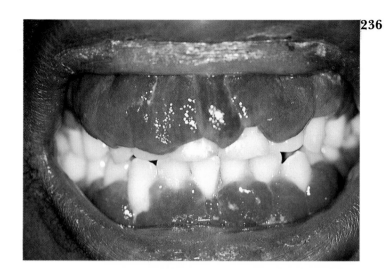

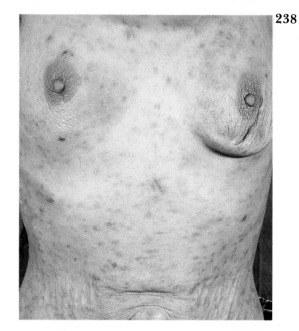

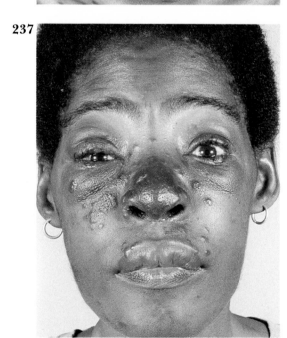

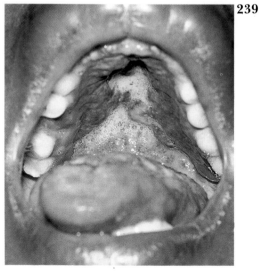

235 & 236 This 28-year-old man has remarkably symmetrical plaques of KS on his face, and uniform infiltration of his gums by tumour tissue, which is rare, although isolated gingival patches or plaques are quite common.

237–239 This young woman has wasting and skin changes suggesting old age, multiple plaques of atypical KS on her swollen face and ulcerated plaques on her palate.

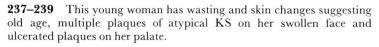

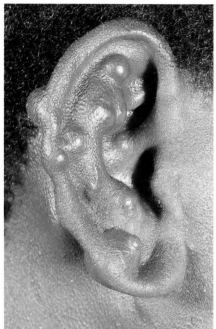

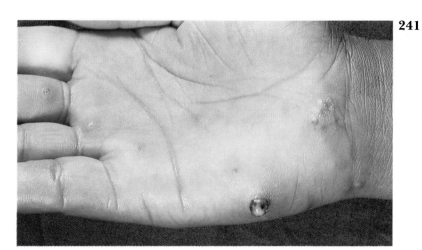

241

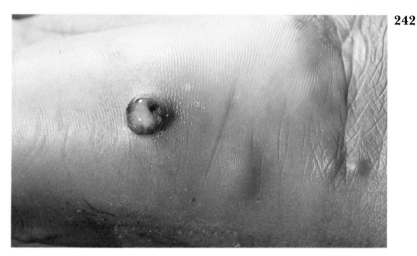

242

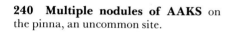

240 Multiple nodules of AAKS on the pinna, an uncommon site.

241 & 242 Kaposi's sarcoma nodules on palm which may be mistaken for granuloma pyogenicum.

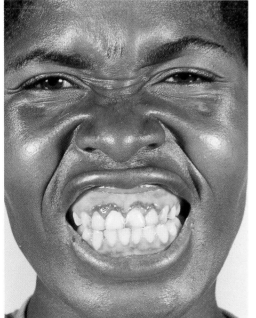

243

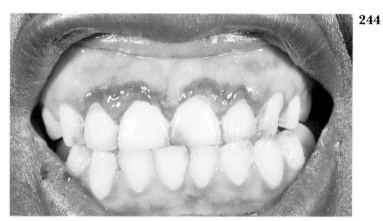

244

243 & 244 Pigmented plaques of atypical Kaposi's sarcoma on face and upper lip. The close-up shows early Kaposi's sarcoma lesions on upper gums.

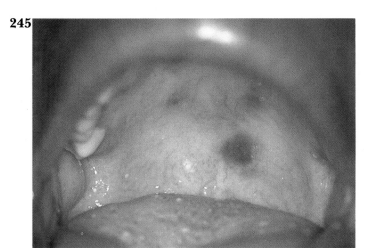

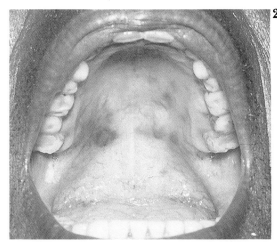

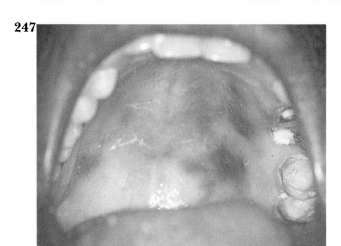

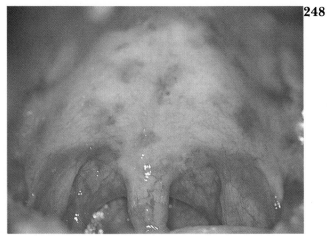

245 Typical early plaques of AAKS on the hard palate.

246 Early plaques of AAKS on the hard palate.

247 This 34-year-old man presented with generalised lymph node enlargement, mild facial swelling and flat patches of Kaposi's sarcoma on his hard palate.

248 Patches of AAKS on the palate and fauces.

249 This woman presented at the age of 37 with enlargement of lymph nodes. She had flat patches of KS in her gums and endoscopy demonstrated nodules of KS in her upper gastrointestinal tract which did not regress during chemotherapy.

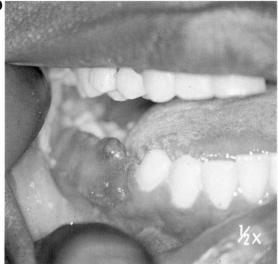

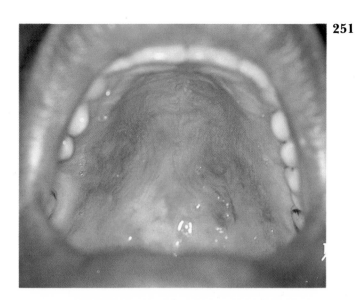

250 A nodule of AAKS on the gingiva.

251 Flat Kaposi's sarcoma on the hard palate in characteristic sites.

252 Stains and plaques of Kaposi's sarcoma on the hard palate.

253 Ulcerated nodules of Kaposi's sarcoma coated with thrush, which also coats the tongue.

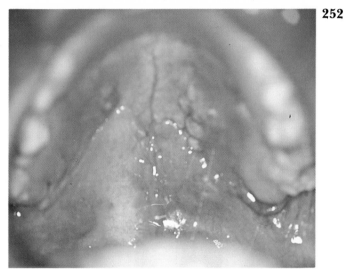

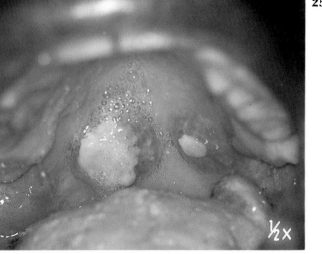

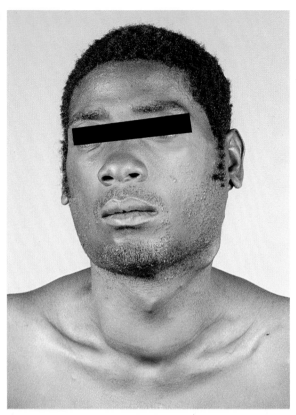

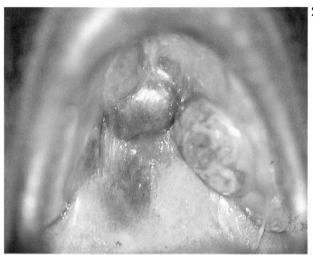

254 & 255 Weight loss, lymph node enlargement and an incidental goitre in a patient with ulcerated nodular Kaposi's sarcoma on his hard palate.

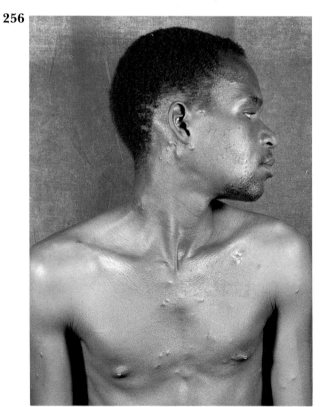

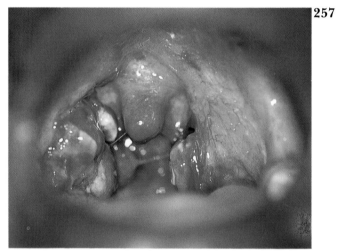

256 & 257 This patient had lost weight and had small skin lesions in a characteristic pattern behind and below the pinna, and on his trunk. He had massive enlargement of both tonsils with visible tumour on their surface and oedema and congestion of the uvula and soft palate.

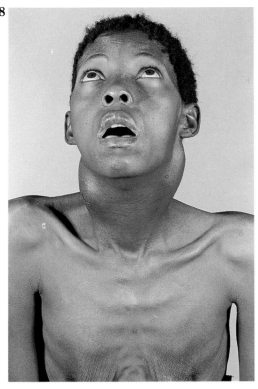

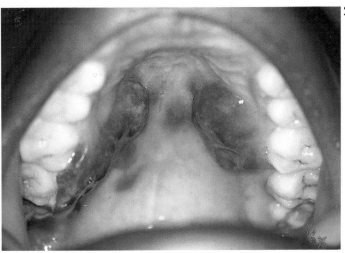

258 & 259 A 27-year-old woman presented with pulmonary tuberculosis and Kaposi's sarcoma. She had irregular ulcerated masses of tumour at characteristic sites on the hard palate and gums. and symmetrical lymphadenopathy.

260 & 261 A man aged 37, presented in December 1983 with a few plaques of KS on his trunk, and small lesions on his tongue. By April 1984 the lesions on the tongue had ulcerated and enlarged in area and depth. Candida is superimposed upon the nodular KS.

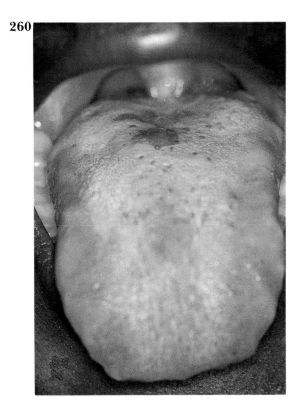

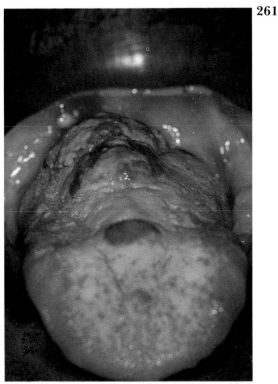

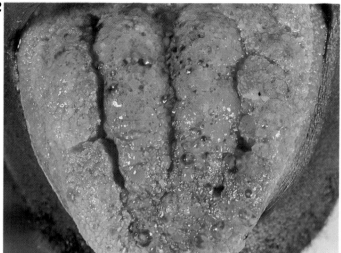

262 This young man presented with a history of vascular lesions of AAKS on his tongue which bled frequently. He had generalised lymphadenopathy and his serology test was positive for HIV.

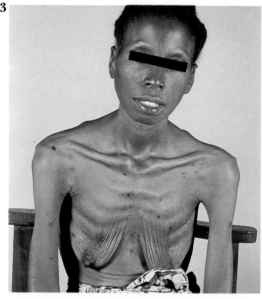

263–269 This woman presented with symmetrical nodular plaques on the tongue with flat KS on the hard palate, before treatment and one month later, showing partial regression following one course of chemotherapy. The plaque is less nodular, less raised and paler in colour. Oral candida has, however, increased in severity. Pictures **264, 266** and **268** were taken before treatment, and **265, 267** and **269** after.

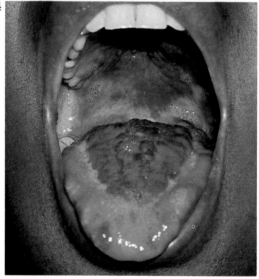

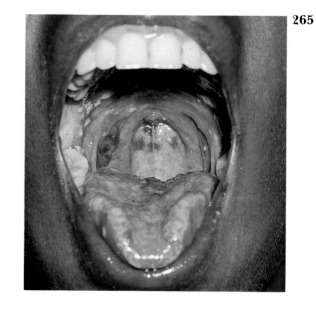

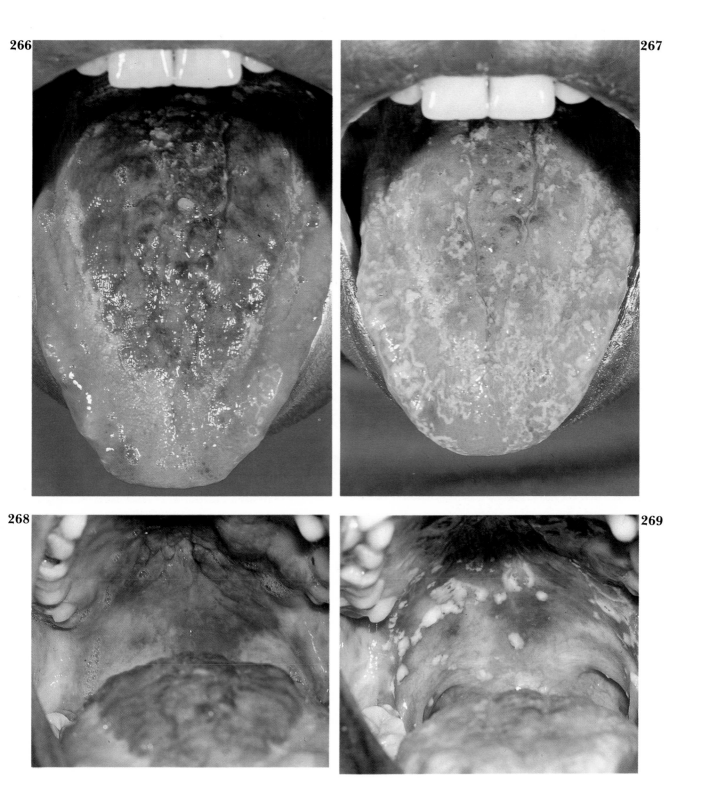

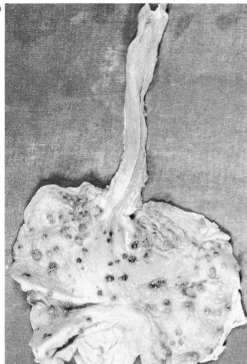

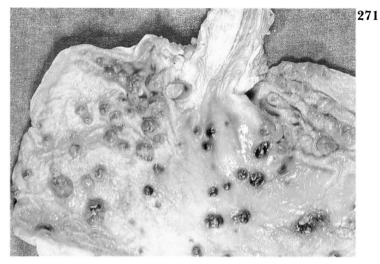

270 **Tumour nodules** in the stomach of a child who died quickly of AAKS.

271 Close-up view of 270.

272 A young woman presented with intestinal obstruction due to ileo-ileal intussusception of the gut which was studded with nodules of Kaposi's sarcoma (resected specimen).

273 **Submucosal nodules of KS** in the colon.

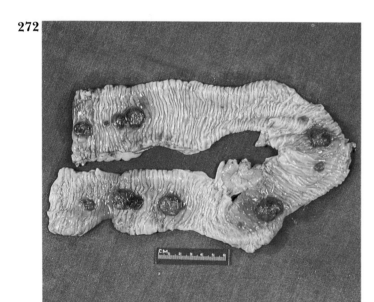

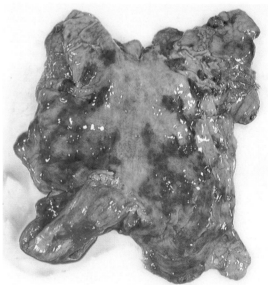

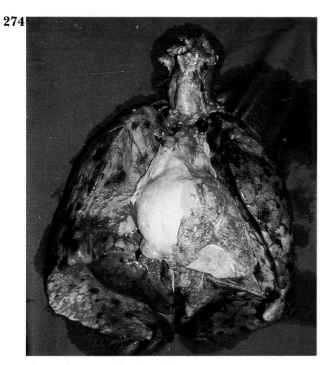
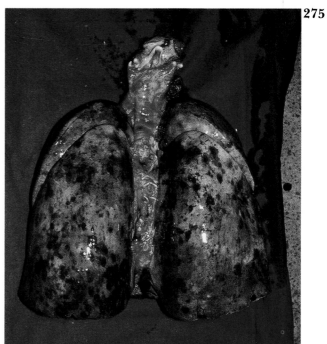

274 & 275   AAKS of both lungs.

The following autopsy case illustrates the multisystem involvement of AAKS.

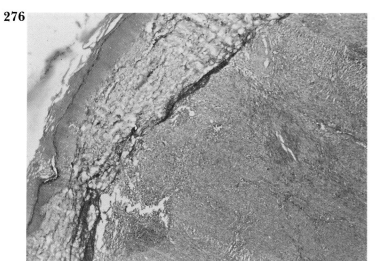

276   Subcutaneous KS

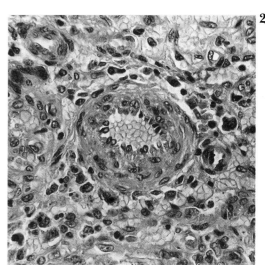

277   Histology of KS

278

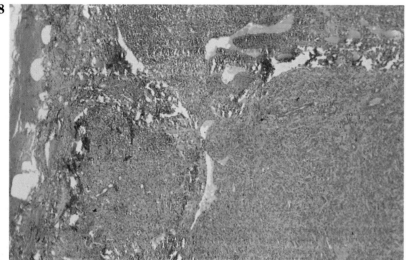

278 KS in the lymph node

279

279 KS in the capsule of the lymph node

280

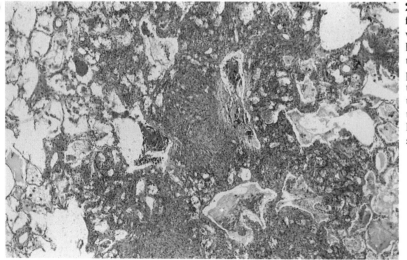

280 Kaposi's sarcoma in the lung from an African man aged 30 years who was HIV positive. One year before death he presented with a few KS nodules on the skin of the legs which rapidly progressed to involve the entire skin of the body, lymph nodes, gastro-intestinal tract from mouth to anus but worse in the stomach, lungs, liver, pancreas and kidneys. Low power view of one of the small KS nodules in the lung.

281 High power of the same lesion.
On the left it shows an alveolus filled
with pigment-laden macrophages, the
alveolar septae are imperceptibly
merging with the KS lesion.

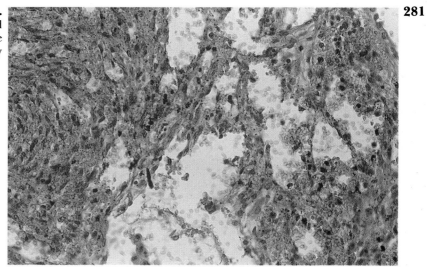

282 KS on the adventitia of the
pulmonary trunk.

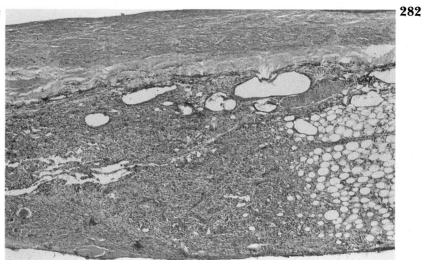

283 KS on the adventitia of the aorta.

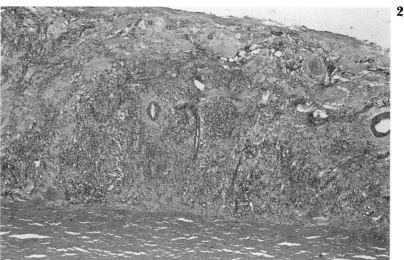

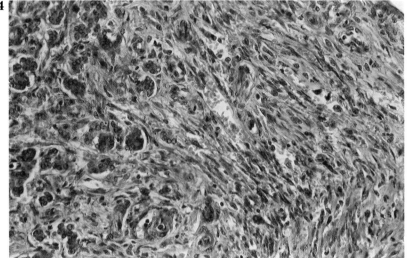

284 KS invading the pancreas.

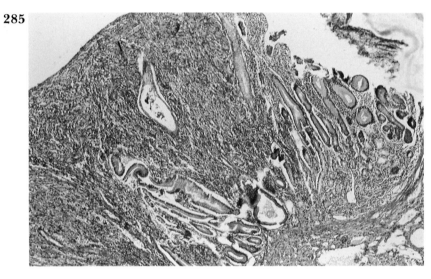

285 KS in the large bowel mucosa.

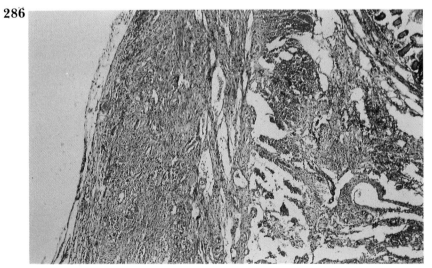

286 **Section of a KS nodule** removed from the peritoneum.

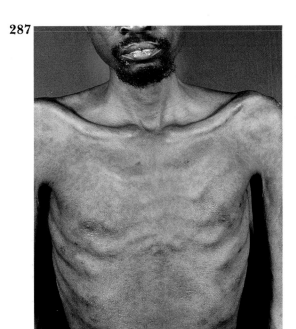

287

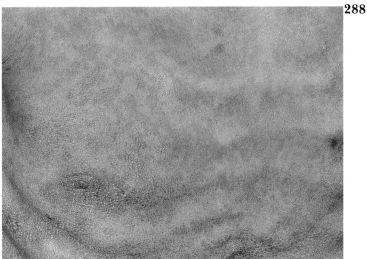

288

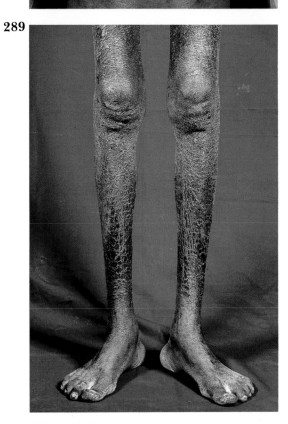

289

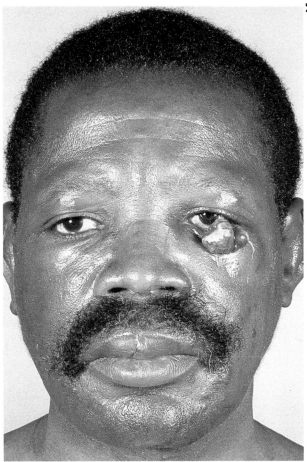

290

287–289 Note the absence of the peripheral skin lesions, confluent patches of purple KS tissue in the skin of the trunk, and gross emaciation. He had HIV positive AAKS.

290 Kaposi's sarcoma of the eyelid has been seen only in patients with AAKS. This lesion regressed completely during treatment.

291

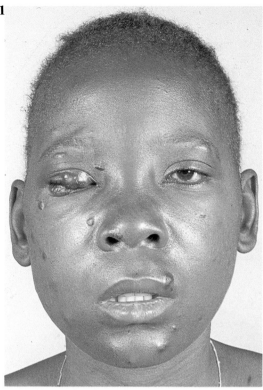

292

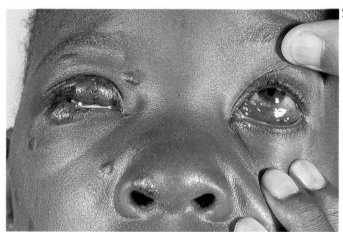

291 & 292   In AAKS plaques on the face are common, less often affecting the eyelids and conjunctiva.

293

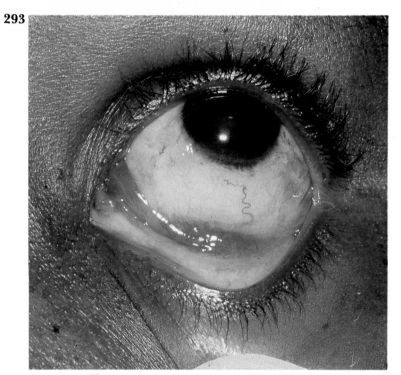

293   Early lesions of atypical KS on the conjunctiva. Patient did not have mucosal or cutaneous lesions of KS.

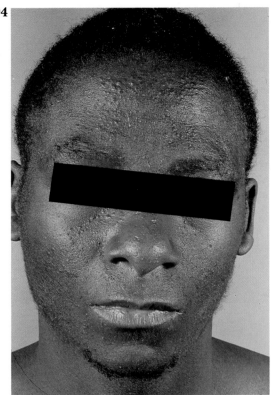

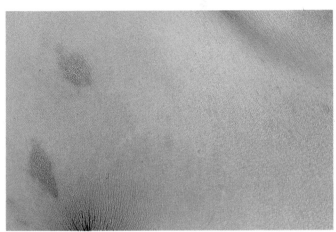

294–296 Papular dermatosis and almost flat skin lesions (KS) in a man with gastrointestinal and lung involvement, AAKS, and encephalopathy.

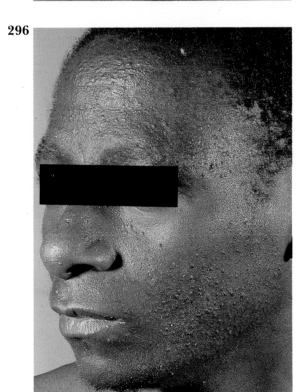

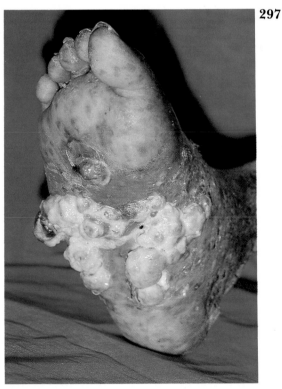

297 Florid tumours of endemic Kaposi's sarcoma.

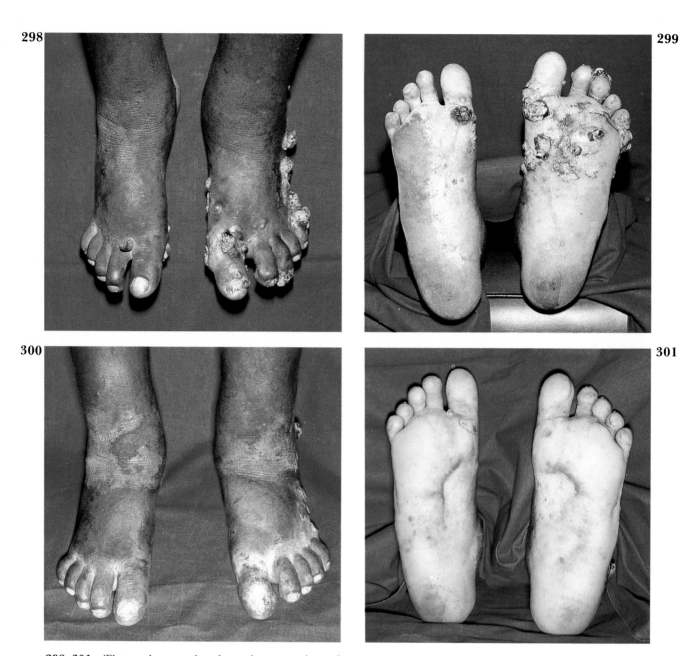

298–301 These photographs show the regression of endemic KS during chemotherapy, and are separated by 9 months.

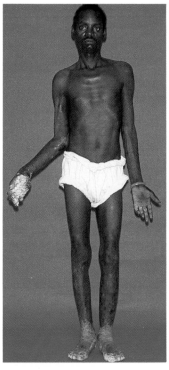
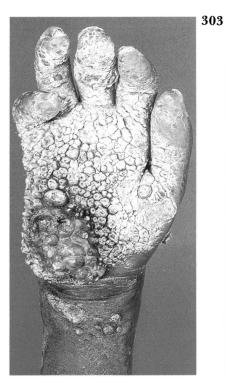
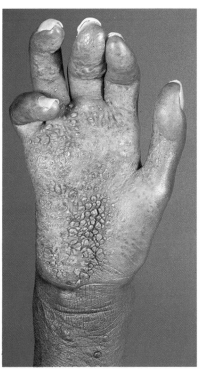

302–304 This 47-year-old man had a 7 year history of nodular swelling on his extremities. His right hand was ulcerated, immobile and grossly enlarged, but even at this site the tumour showed an excellent response to chemotherapy over a period of four months.

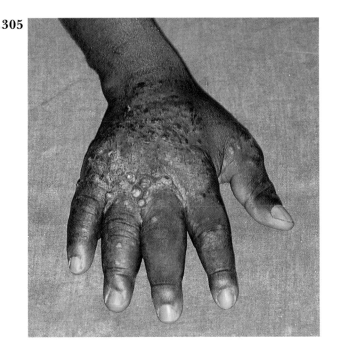
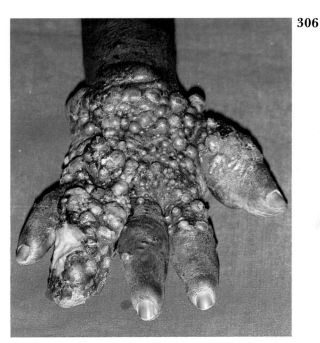

305 & 306 Endemic Kaposi's sarcoma restricted to one hand. The first photograph was taken in September 1984 and the second in July 1987 when the tumour had become resistant to all available cytotoxic agents. An amputation was done.

307

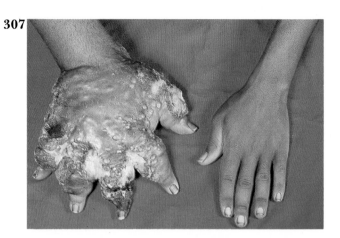

308

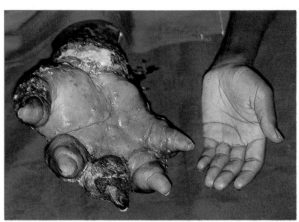

309

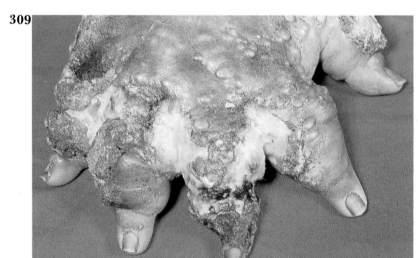

307–310 This patient insisted that his symptoms started only four months before these photographs were taken. His left hand is normal, the right hand displays a florid and infiltrative tumour, which has cut off the blood supply to his now gangrenous middle finger.

310

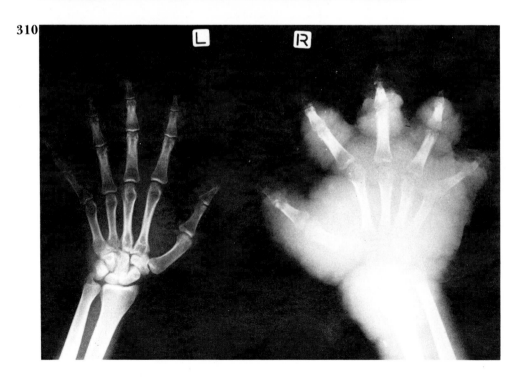

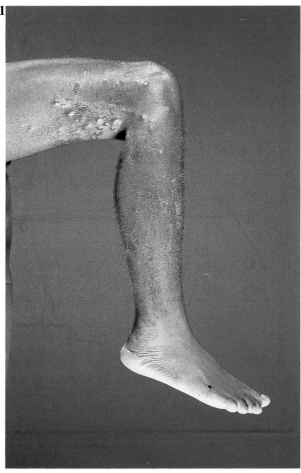

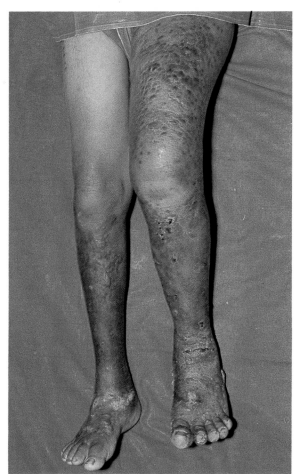

311 Long-standing infiltration of endemic Kaposi's sarcoma around joints leads to contractures. Successful chemotherapy was followed by almost complete recovery of knee extension from the 90 degrees contracture shown in this photograph.

312 An elderly woman had endemic Kaposi's sarcoma. There is widespread thickening and hyperpigmentation due to nearly confluent lesions, causing a flexion contraction of the left knee and swelling of the left leg.

313 A boy aged 10 years presented with masses in the abdomen, thrombocytopoenia and this hairy, naevus-like plaque on his back which was Kaposi's sarcoma. He responded poorly to chemotherapy but was seen before HIV-related Kaposi's sarcoma was recognised in Zambia.

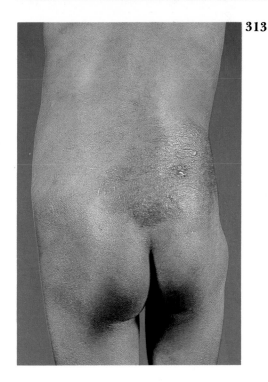

Section 11: Slim Disease

Slim disease is the name given to a new syndrome, which appeared in 1982, by inhabitants of the Rakai district in South Western Uganda. Patients present with fever, an itchy maculo-papular rash, prolonged diarrhoea and progressive severe weight loss. In Rakai 100% of patients with slim disease were seropositive for antibodies to HIV and it appears to be the same entity as enteropathic AIDS described in Zaire and Tanzania.

The diarrhoea is watery, rarely contains obvious blood and occurs in episodes lasting days or weeks. It is not continuous, at least at first. Careful examination of stools or rectal biopsies shows either Cryptosporidium or Isospora belli in most patients, but other more conventional pathogens, such as Entamoeba histolytica or Giardia are rarely found.

Slim disease is a useful term for patients whose dominant symptoms are the triad of diarrhoea, severe wasting and an itchy rash, provided that clinicians exclude treatable causes of diarrhoea and provide supportive care to exploit the natural remissions which may interrupt a generally downhill clinical course.

Overcrowded towns with poor sanitation may favour the spread of opportunist enteric pathogens and be responsible for the varying incidence of slim disease in tropical communities which have similar seropositivity rates.

Differential diagnoses:

1. Chronic enteric infections—bacillary dysentery, bacterial agents like Salmonella, Streptococci, fungi, viral and tuberculous infection.

2. Parasitic causes
   Protozoa—amoebic colitis, giardiasis, Leishmania donovani
   Helminths—Strongyloides

3. Malabsorption—primary and secondary malabsorption syndromes.

4. Nutritional diseases such as protein energy malnutrition in children and pellagra.

5. Malignancies.

6. Chronic illnesses such as trypanosomiasis.

314
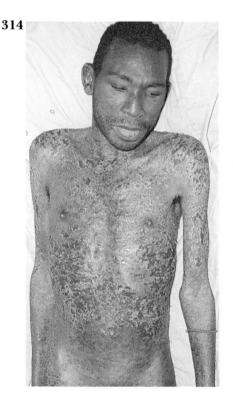

315
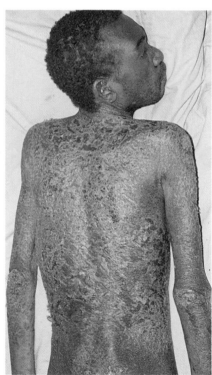

314 & 315 This young man with AIDS presented with a history of recurrent diarrhoea and weight loss. Physical examination revealed pellagrous skin changes, generalised lymphadenopathy and buccal candidiasis.

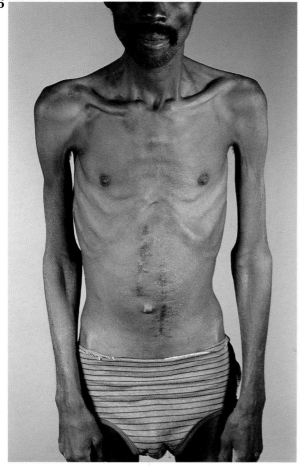

316

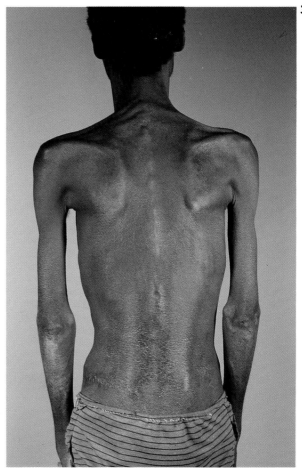

317

316 & 317   Slim disease: chronic diarrhoea with gross weight loss in a patient with AIDS. The skin shows papular dermatosis with atrophic scars.

318   Cryptosporidium in the stool of an HIV-infected patient with chronic diarrhoea and wasting.

318

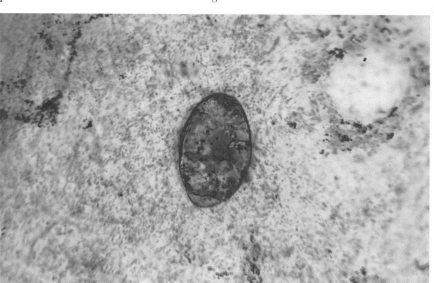

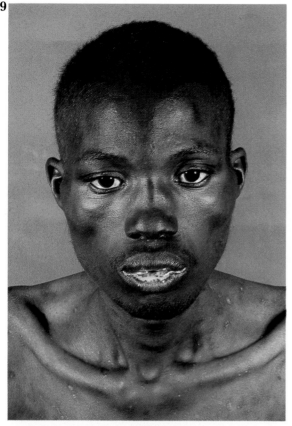

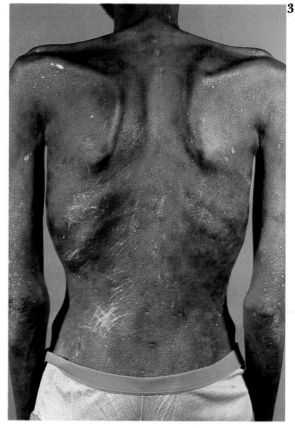

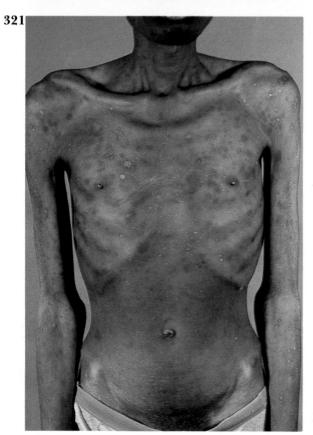

319–321 **Slim disease** with pellagrous skin changes.

Section 12: Pulmonary Manifestation of AIDS

In the Northern hemisphere Pneumocystis carinii is the commonest opportunist pathogen infecting the lungs of AIDS patients, but it does not appear to be as common a cause of respiratory symptoms or pneumonia in the tropics. Respiratory symptoms with or without abnormal chest radiographs are, however, common.

Lobar pneumonia presents with classical symptoms and signs in patients with symptomatic HIV infections and usually shows the classic radiologic signs. Resolution following appropriate antibiotic treatment is complete but may take longer than usual.

Mycobacterium tuberculosis is being recognised as the commonest opportunist pathogen of AIDS patients in the tropics, where extra-pulmonary lesions are particularly common. In the chest unilateral pleural effusion, cavitating apical disease and miliary tuberculosis are seen, but less typical lesions may occur alone, or in combination with other diseases, such as pulmonary Kaposi's sarcoma. Several studies have shown that between 40 and 60% of patients with newly-diagnosed tuberculosis are seropositive for HIV antibodies. Tuberculosis control programmes in some countries are reporting increasing numbers of new cases since 1985.

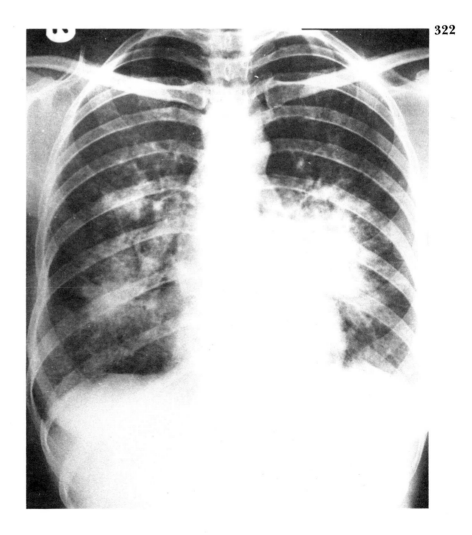

322 Pneumocystis carinii pneumonia.

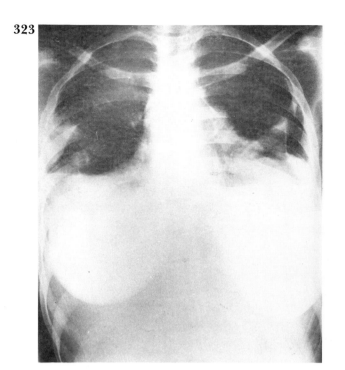

323 Bilateral tubercular pleural effusion.

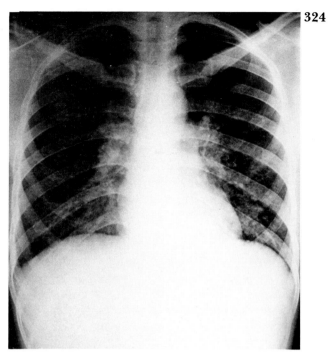

324 & 325 Miliary tuberculosis in patients with AIDS.

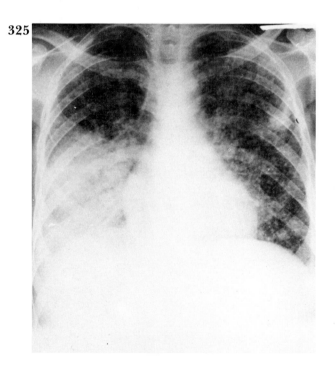

326 Pulmonary tuberculosis in a patient with AIDS.

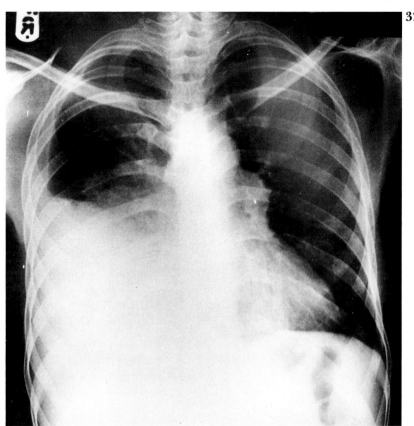

327 & 328 This 32-year-old man presented with AAKS and a unilateral pleural effusion which decreased in volume during 10 weeks treatment with cytotoxic drugs.

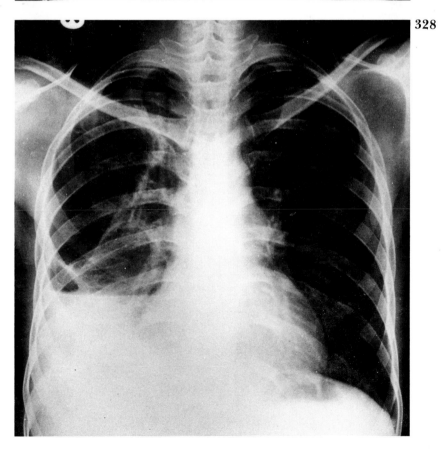

329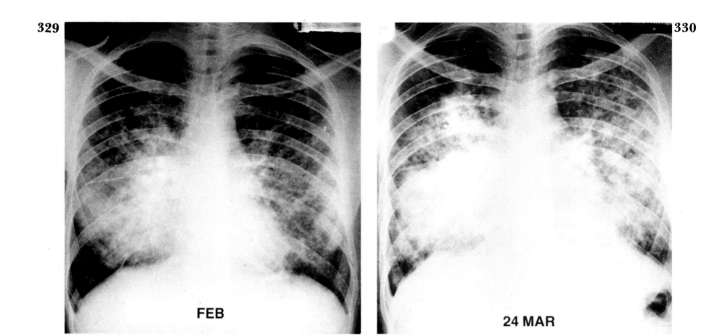

FEB

24 MAR

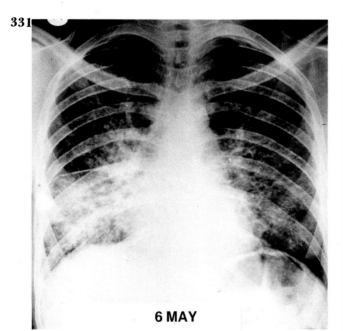

6 MAY

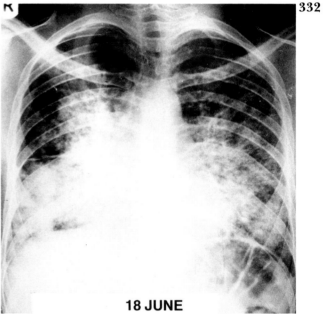

18 JUNE

329–332 This young man had cough, fever, dyspnoea and haemoptysis late in 1982. A presumptive diagnosis of pulmonary tuberculosis was made and appropriate therapy started, but his symptoms worsened and his chest radiograph showed more extensive infiltration between February and March 1983, when a diagnosis of AAKS was made on the basis of skin lesions. In April and May he received chemotherapy and symptoms and signs improved for a short period. The final radiograph shows increasing infiltration again as dyspnoea returned before his death due to AAKS.

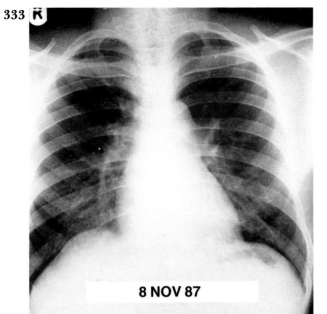

333

8 NOV 87

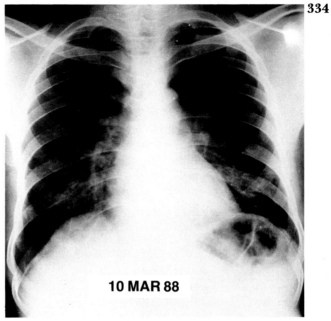

334

10 MAR 88

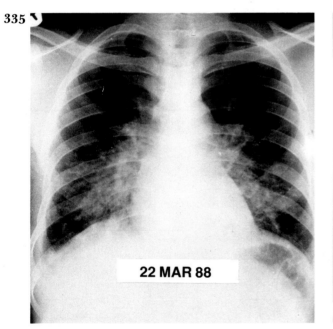

335

22 MAR 88

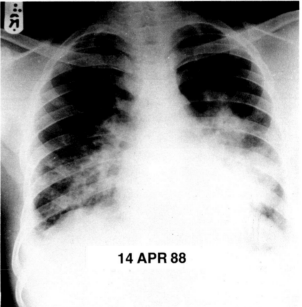

336

14 APR 88

333–336 Sequential radiographs of a patient treated for AAKS in 1987 who developed fever, chest pain and cough in March 1988 These symptoms did not respond to antibiotic therapy and new plaques of KS appeared on his face and palate as chest radiographs showed increasing perihilar and basal infiltrations.

In the tropics patients who complain of cough, haemoptyses and weight loss frequently have pulmonary tuberculosis and this diagnosis is likely to be assumed even when sputum examination fails to show acid and alcohol fast bacilli (AAFB). In some HIV-infected patients with these symptoms chest radiographs show a fluffy infiltrate in the perihilar and lower zones, which is nearly symmetrical with little or no pathology at the apices and (usually) no pleural effusion. Examination of the mouth might show typical patches or plaques of Kaposi's sarcoma.

In children recurrent respiratory tract infections such as tonsillitis, pharyngo-otitis media and pneumonia occur frequently. Of the serious infections pulmonary tuberculosis is very common amongst all age groups. Pleural effusion is sometimes tuberculous in origin but some may be "sympathetic". Lymphoid interstitial pneumonia is seen in children and may be difficult to distinguish from other pneumoniae.

Drug reactions are common especially in those patients receiving anti-tuberculosis drugs. These range from a maculopapular rash to vesiculo-bullous eruptions sometimes in association with oral ulceration and gastro-intestinal symptoms (Stevens-Johnson Syndrome).

Pericardial effusions occur less often but these have a bad prognosis.

Differential diagnoses:

Tuberculosis without HIV-I infection

The clinical manifestations with or without HIV infection are the same.

Pulmonary fungal infection

In the areas where histoplasmosis and coccidiodiomycosis occur these should be kept in mind. Pulmonary candidiasis should also be excluded.

Carcinoma of the lung

This occurs in men and women in their 4th to 7th decades of life.

Inhaled foreign body especially in children

This may cause collapse of a segment of a lung and an unresolving pneumonia.

Tracheo-oesophageal fistula in children

Persistent aspiration leads to unresolving pneumonia.

Section 13: Sepsis

As a general rule non-urgent surgery should be avoided in patients who are HIV seropositive. The stress of surgery may alter the balance between the patient and his retrovirus infection, leading to deterioration. Some HIV patients deteriorate rapidly after major surgery without any other detectable cause.

Surgical sepsis

Surgeons are trained to exclude diabetes mellitus whenever they see a patient with sepsis, but now, in the tropics, they should also look for signs of HIV-disease and, if these are found, test blood for HIV antibodies.

Infection that should be easily localised is sometimes not localised. Fournier's gangrene and necrotising fasciitis have been found in association with HIV disease, as have recurrent and multiple subcutaneous abscesses.

Tropical ulcers may appear on the lower limbs of HIV patients with no other detectable cause and fail to heal with standard therapy but instead, enlarge slowly over several months. Limb gangrene may also appear for no apparent reason in young people, and severe pelvic inflammatory disease is common. In many HIV-I patients weight loss, scars of multidermatomal herpes zoster, generalised lymphadenopathy, oral candidiasis, or other opportunist infections provides supporting evidence for the underlying HIV infection.

Orthopaedic complications associated with HIV disease includes septic arthritis and septic complications of internal fixation. In high seroprevalence areas HIV testing should be done before internal fixation. The stress of both the operation and the infection may hasten deterioration of the patient's immunity.

In the absence of underlying anaemia or gross infection, skin grafts normally take successfully in HIV positive patients.

Surgical tuberculosis in HIV-I patients is common. Lymph node masses are asymmetric, large and often partly fluctuant. Tuberculous lymph nodes in the abdomen are more likely to be retroperitoneal than mesenteric, although disease in both sites is seen. Histological examination of tuberculous lymph nodes shows numerous acid and alcohol fast bacilli (AAFB) when appropriate stains are used. Giant cells and a granulomatous reaction are often absent in HIV-related tuberculous adenitis. Adult patients who have stable spinal deformities following childhood tuberculosis may develop paraparesis progressing to paraplegia as immune competence wanes.

Cutaneous sepsis

This may present as recurrent furunculosis, impetigo contagiosum, impetigo bullosum (seen in infants), echthyma, streptococcal acrodermatitis, otitis externa, erysipelas, cellulitis and tropical ulcers.

Pelvic inflammatory disease (PID)

This is the most significant genital complication of HIV-I infection in the female. It is caused by spread of infection from the cervix to the upper genital tract. Causative organisms include Neisseria gonorrhoeae, Chlamydia trachomatis, and Mycoplasma hominis. Secondary infection with other organisms, especially Gram negative rods and anaerobes, which are normal residents in the vagina, vulva and bowel, results in acute tubo-ovarian sepsis and peritonitis.

PID is suggested by a history of lower abdominal pain, malaise, vaginal discharge and dyspareunia or dysmenorrhoea. On examination findings are of fever, abdominal tenderness, adnexal tenderness or mass, pain on movement of the cervix and a purulent cervical discharge. Recurrent episodes of PID cause infertility and predispose to ectopic pregnancy. Rupture of a pyosalpinx or tubo-ovarian abscess causes peritonitis, septicaemia, and shock with high mortality.

Epidemiologic factors which increase the risk of PID include promiscuous sexual relationships, use of intrauterine contraceptive devices, minor gynaecological operations and immunosuppression caused by HIV.

There is an association between HIV infection and severe female genital tract sepsis, including both pelvic inflammatory disease and pregnancy related infection. If infection is treated promptly some HIV patients heal similarly to HIV negative patients. How labour is to be managed is an issue yet to be resolved but it appears that Caesarean section, particularly in prolonged labour can be complicated by severe uterine infection which may require hysterectomy.

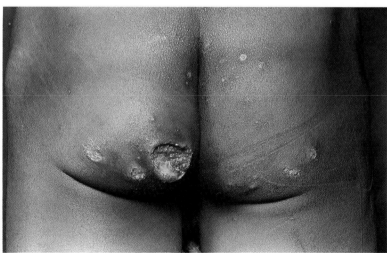

337

337 Furunculosis leading to ecthyma in a patient with AIDS-related complex. Response to antibiotics is slow.

Other diseases normally predisposing to sepsis may also be present in an HIV-I infected patient, including diabetes mellitus, chronic malnutrition, sickle cell anaemia, congenital immunodeficiencies, malignancy, prematurity, severe malaria and those who have had a splenectomy or are receiving cytotoxic drugs.

The differential diagnosis of patients with septic conditions depends upon the mode of presentation. For example, if a patient presents with a chronic leg ulcer the differential diagnosis includes sickle cell disease, tropical, acute infection, trauma, squamous carcinoma, septicaemia, and bacterial endocarditis.

Venous stasis and arterial insufficiency are uncommon in the tropics although their incidence is increasing, particularly in the cities.

The differential diagnosis of prolonged postsurgical fever depends upon the operation performed but includes chest, wound or deep seated infection, peritonitis, urinary tract infection, malaria, drug hypersensitivity, and septicaemia. Tuberculosis, connective tissue disorders, undiagnosed malignancy, drug reactions, ENT, meningeal, bone and joint sepsis must be excluded in pyrexia of unknown origin.

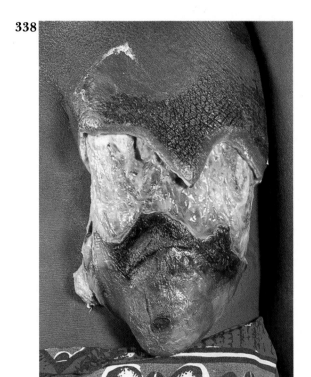

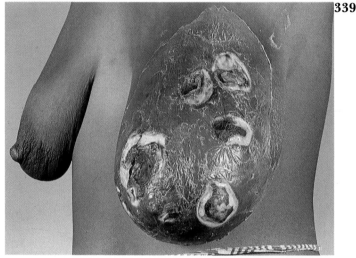

338 Young patient with AIDS developed cellulitis of left breast which sloughed despite antibiotic therapy.

339 Twenty-two year old patient developed multiple abscesses on left breast following delivery. Abscesses burst open leaving behind discharging sinuses. She had generalised lymphadenopathy and purulent vaginal discharge. Her serology test was positive.

340–342 HIV-positive man with no local or systemic pathology to account for ulcers on both feet. Over five months the ulcers enlarged despite conventional care by elevation and local cleaning. Sloughs were so slow to separate that surgical debridement was done, but granulations capable of supporting skin graft have not developed. Note weight loss during period of observation.

340

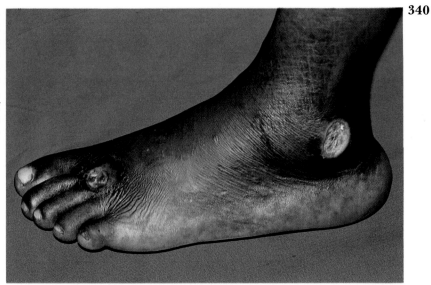

341

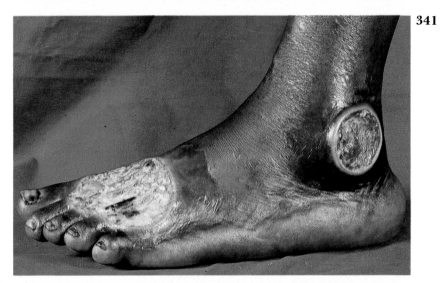

342

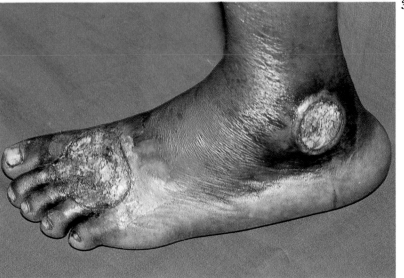

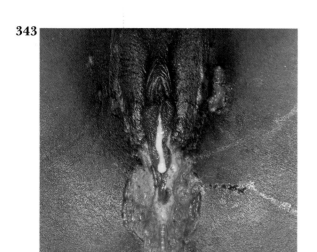

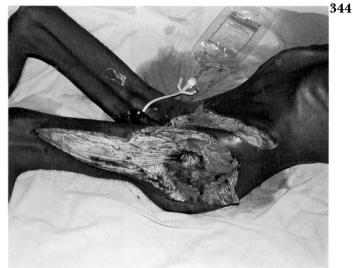

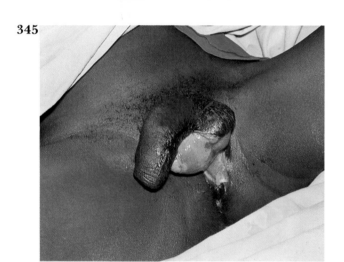

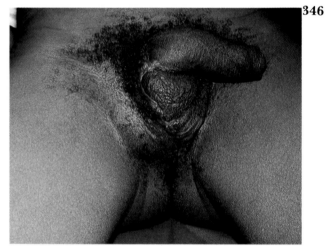

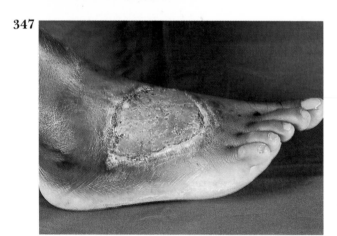

343 This HIV-positive patient suffered extensive perianal skin loss due to infection.

344 15-year-old boy who presented with osteomyelitis of the proximal femur. Despite sequestrectomy and multiple drainage his wounds failed to heal and he required extensive debridement for necrotising fasciitis.

345 & 346 This HIV-positive patient developed Fournier's gangrene. Good wound care and split skin grafting resulted in complete healing despite his HIV status.

347 **Unexplained skin ulceration** in unusual sites has been observed in some HIV-positive patients. This woman has had a split skin graft to a non-traumatic ulcer on the dorsum of her foot.

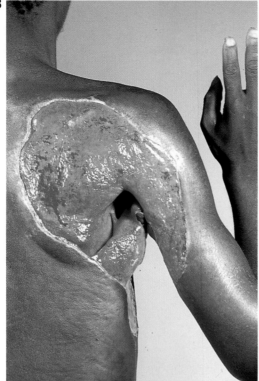

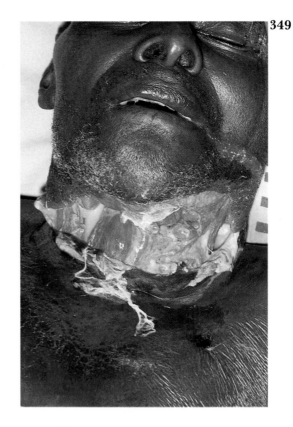

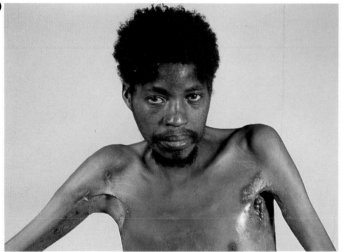

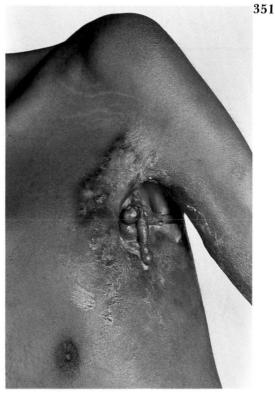

348 **Extensive tissue necrosis** following axillary lymph node infection in HIV positive patient.

349 Patient with HIV disease developed a furuncle on the neck which progressed to extensive soft tissue necrosis (cancrum syndrome).

350 & 351 **Scrofuloderma** from underlying tuberculous lymph nodes in a patient with AIDS.

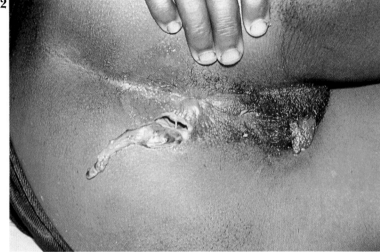

352   **Perianal fistula** discharging pus in a patient with AIDS.

353   **Recurrent pyomyositis** in a patient infected with HIV.

354   **Open wound** following drainage of septic arthritis of the knee in a 23-year-old male. A number of young adults with septic arthritis have been found to be HIV positive. Since septic arthritis is unusual in this age group acquired immuno-deficiency appears to be implicated.

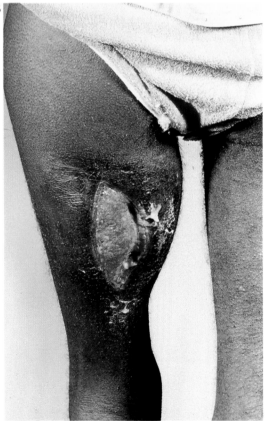

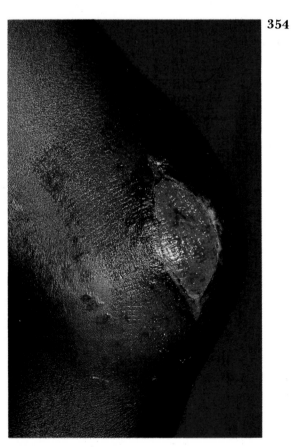

355 A lymphogranuloma venereum ulcer on the vulva.

356 Severe necrotising fasciitis requiring widespread excision of skin and subcutaneous tissue over abdomen and back. The initial septic focus was an ulcer on the vulva.

357–359 Open laparotomy wound following peritoneal sepsis due to ruptured tubo-ovarian abscess. This patient was HIV positive. The follow-up photograph 16 days later showed that the wound was healing despite underlying anaemia. At 6 months the wound was perfectly healed and the patient fit and well without clinical signs of HIV disease.

355

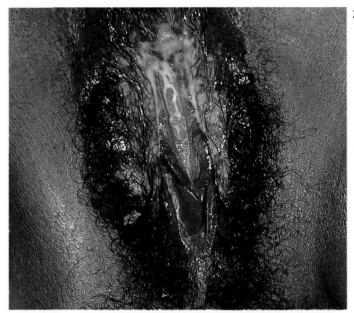

356

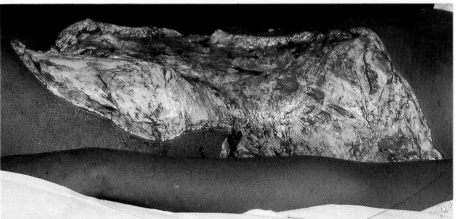

357   **358**   **359**

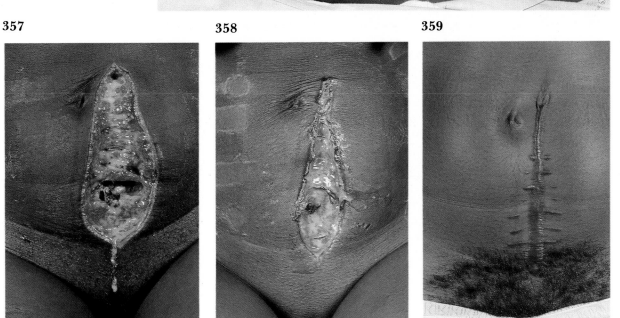

360

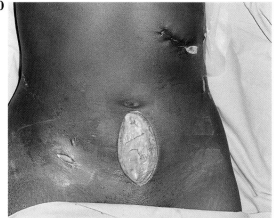

360–362 Laparotomy wound following severe peritonitis due to septic abortion in a HIV positive patient. A left subphrenic abscess has also been drained. Erect chest x-ray of the same patient showing her left subphrenic abscess which developed ten days after laparotomy. Her left subphrenic abscess was later complicated by empyema. Although the pleural cavity was drained and she was discharged, she died at home 4 months after her initial presentation with chronic sepsis.

363 & 364 19-year-old HIV positive woman mechanically ventilated after laparotomy and hysterectomy for peritonitis secondary to criminal abortion. The first chest radiograph was taken on admission to intensive care. The second, three days later when her right lung was obliterated. She died shortly afterwards.

361

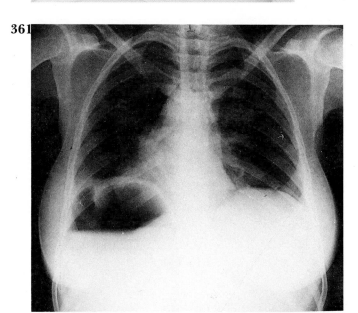

362

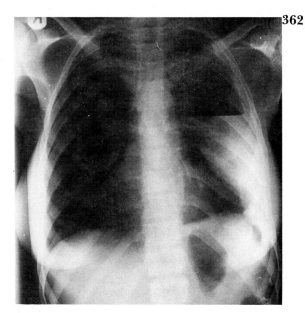

363

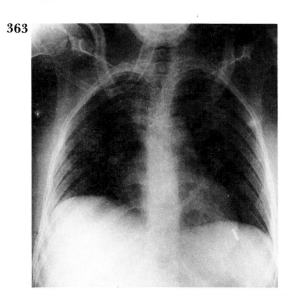

364

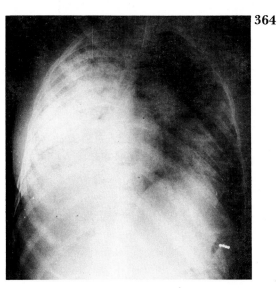

Section 14: Diseases of the Nervous System

Neurological disease is caused by the HIV, directly by infection of nerve tissue or by opportunistic infections and tumours. The main neurological disorders are dementia, neuropathy, myelopathy, retinitis, meningitis and focal neurological disease. Neurological disorders may occur during the early stages of HIV infection.

Dementia

HIV-I and possibly cytomegalovirus cause dementia in more than 50% of African AIDS patients. It varies from a subtle slowing of mental and motor function to a state of apathy characterized by withdrawal, short term memory loss, poor concentration and difficulty making simple calculations (serial sevens). In the later stages disorientation, confusion, incontinence and seizures may occur. However, most patients remain conscious and aware of their surroundings. AIDS dementia is frequently accompanied by abnormal neurological signs—frontal lobe release signs, ataxia, neuropathy and myelopathy.

Description of frontal lobe release signs

Snout and palmomental reflexes are present in most African AIDS patients. The snout reflex is elicited by pressing or tapping lightly with a knuckle or tendon hammer on closed lips. In positive cases this will cause a contraction of the lips giving the appearance of a snout. The palmomental reflex is elicited by stroking the palm of the hand near the thenar eminence with a key. In positive cases this will result in a brief contraction of the ipsilateral mentalis muscle which causes a puckering of the chin. The grasp reflex is absent.

Neuropathy

Main cause: HIV-I
Severe generalized muscle wasting is present in almost all African AIDS patients. A distal symmetrical polyneuropathy is found in approximately one quarter of patients at the time of diagnosis. Reflexes are typically depressed.

Myelopathy

Main cause: HIV-I, Mycobacteriae.
Ataxia, tremor, hyperreflexia, and positive Babinski signs are to be found in a number of AIDS patients. They occur mainly as isolated findings and in dementia. Spastic paraparesis may occur in the disease in a few cases. Nearly all male patients are impotent early in the disease.

Retinitis

Main causes: cytomegalovirus, toxoplasmosis, and HIV-I.
The findings of retinitis in the clinical setting of AIDS in the absence of other known causes is virtually diagnostic of AIDS. Cotton wool exudates are found in about one fifth of AIDS patients and flame shaped and punctate haemorrhages also occur, but less frequently. Rarely, a severe vasculitis may result in blindness.

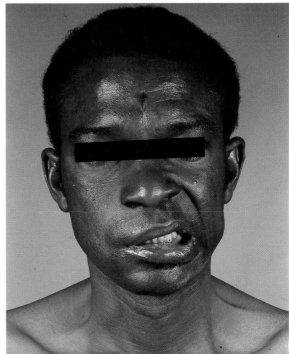

365

365 Isolated mononeuropathy of a cranial nerve or peripheral nerve occurs in some HIV-infected patients and may resolve spontaneously.

Meningitis

Main causes: Cryptococcus, Mycobacteria.
Meningitis in AIDS has been found more frequently in some areas of Africa (eg. Zaire) than in others. The presence of persistent headache, fever, vomiting with or without meningeal signs suggest meningitis: acute symptoms are rare. Special stains - acid fast stain (Mycobacteria) and India ink preparation (Cryptococcus) are necessary to detect the organisms in cerebrospinal fluid.

Focal disease

Main causes: Toxoplasma, lymphoma, tuberculoma.

AIDS is not usually characterized by focal neurological disease but hemiparesis, cranial nerve palsies, mononeuritis and multiple seizures do occur, though infrequently. Toxoplasmosis appears to be uncommon in African patients with HIV-I infections.

Pre-AIDS neurological disease

Main causes: HIV-I, herpes zoster.
Abnormal neurological features can antedate clinical AIDS. Encephalitis, meningitis, myelitis and polyneuritis may occur at seroconversion or during the latent phase of HIV-I infection. In particular, encephalitis and myelitis can be fatal at this stage.

366
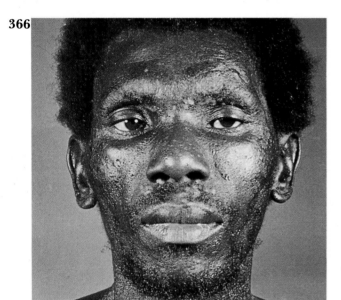

367
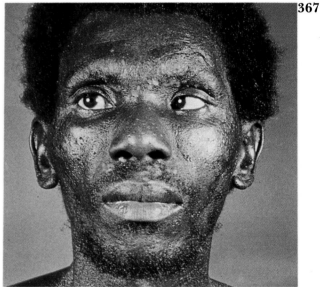

368
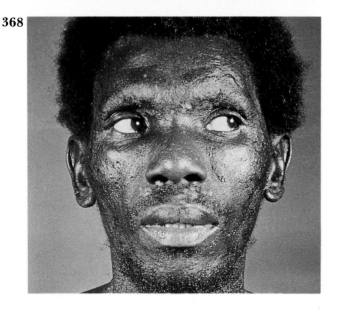

366–368 Paralysis of right lateral rectus muscle of the eye in a patient with HIV-related encephalopathy and seborrhoeic dermatitis.

Section 15: Other Tumours

Atypical Kaposi's sarcoma is the commonest tumour in HIV-I infected patients in the tropics, as elsewhere. An increase in B-cell lymphoma observed in the United States is not yet evident in the tropics.

Several years will be needed to establish causative associations between HIV infections and individual cancers. As well as influencing the multifactorial initiation and promotion of carcinogenesis, HIV infection may influence the age at onset, sex distribution, clinical features and natural history of common cancers. Preliminary observations suggest that the incidence and behaviour of common tumours which are known or suspected to be of viral aetiology may be changing under the influence of HIV.

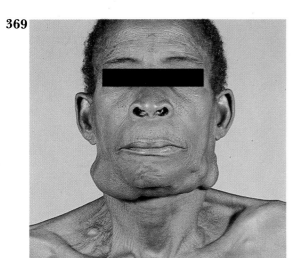
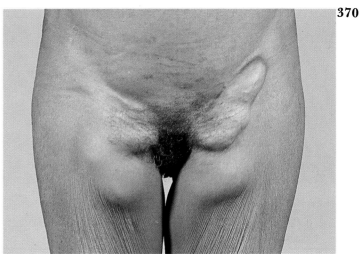

369 & 370   An HIV seropositive patient with non-Hodgkin's lymphoma and weight loss. This association has not been investigated, therefore, HIV infection may be coincidental.

Section 16: Paediatric AIDS

Infants of seropositive mothers

90-95% of infants born of seropositive mothers are seropositive at birth because of placental transfer of IgG. However, those with high levels of IgM in their blood are more likely to be infected, particularly if other congenital infections are excluded. Congenital syphilis must be excluded as some mothers and their infants could have both diseases.

About 50% of the children born to such mothers are seronegative for HIV-I at 1 year and the other half remain seropositive. Amongst HIV seropositive infants, 30-40% die within the first year of life. These infants have repeated episodes of fever, respiratory infections such as otitis media and pneumonias, oropharyngeal candidiasis, diarrhoea and vomiting. These symptoms may lead to protein energy malnutrition. Hepatosplenomegaly, generalised lymphadenopathy, maculopapular dermatosis, herpes zoster and pyogenic skin lesions are some of the features of the disease in children. An appreciable number of children develop pulmonary tuberculosis during the course of the illness despite BCG immunisation. Those who survive the first year of life may develop Kaposi's sarcoma or lymphomas. Encephalitis, meningitis and recurrent Bell's palsy are central nervous system manifestations. The prognosis of those infants who remain seropositive for HIV is poor: most develop AIDS within the first decade of life.

Blood transfusion induced paediatric AIDS

Due to repeated transfusion of unscreened blood and blood products (such as cryoprecipitate), children with sickle cell disease, thalassaemia and haemophilia are at greater risk of acquiring AIDS.

Immunisation of patients with paediatric AIDS

Immunisation with live vaccines does not seem to have any adverse effects in children infected with HIV. However, the efficacy of these vaccines is not known.

Breast feeding and HIV infection

Although it is potentially possible to acquire HIV infection through breast feeding, the risk is epidemiologically insignificant; so breast feeding by mothers who have HIV infection should not be discouraged.

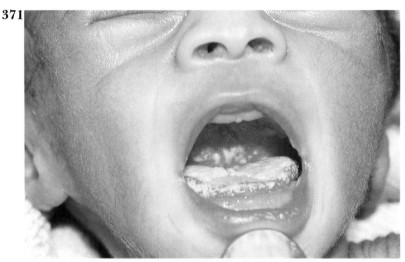

371 A two months old infant born to a mother with AIDS. The child developed pneumonia and oral candidiasis.

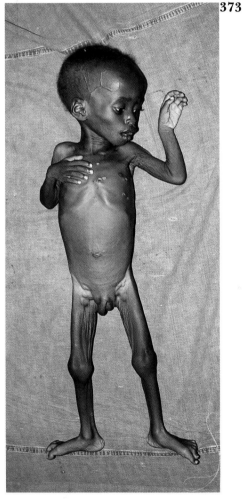

373 This child was first seen at the age of 9 months for recurrent diarrhoea, otitis media and failure to thrive. He was marasmic and had generalised lymphadenopathy, and hepatosplenomegaly. Chest x-ray showed evidence of pulmonary tuberculosis. HIV tests in mother, baby and the father were positive.

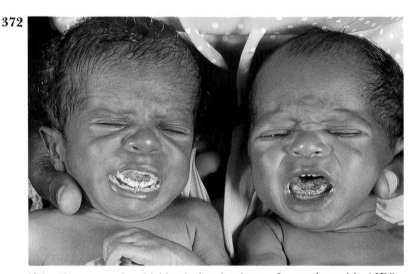

372 Three months old identical twins born of a mother with AIDS. They presented with a history of recurrent respiratory infections and failure to thrive. Examination revealed hepatosplenomegaly and extensive candidiasis.

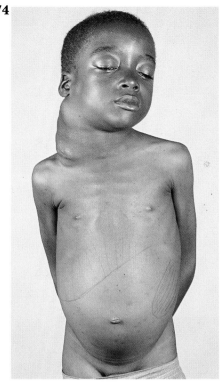

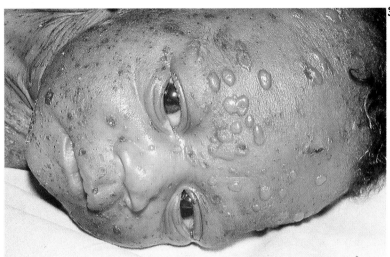

374 A child with huge cervical lymphadenopathy and hepatosplenomegaly with HIV infection.

375 A week old infant with disseminated herpes simplex born to a mother with ARC. The mother had herpes genitalis at the time of vaginal delivery.

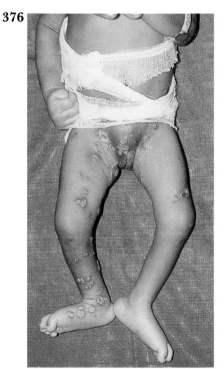

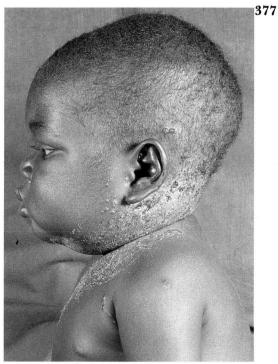

376 An infant with disseminated herpes simplex. Died at the age of 2 weeks. Mother had ARC and herpes genitalis at the time of delivery.

377 Infant born to a mother with ARC. He developed herpes zoster and generalised lymphadenopathy. Herpes zoster is usually a disease of old people.

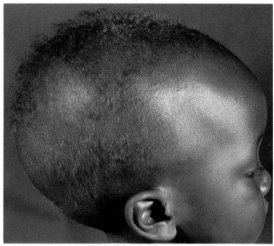

378 Sparse, brittle hair on the scalp in a malnourished patient with ARC. This should be differentiated from hair changes seen with protein energy malnutrition.

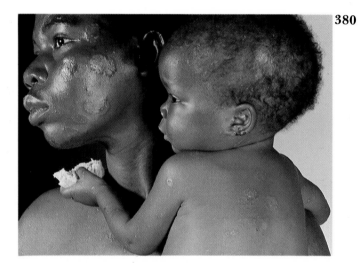

379 & 380 Ten months old infant born to a mother with ARC. Mother and infant had extensive lesions of tinea corporis and pruritic papular dermatosis.

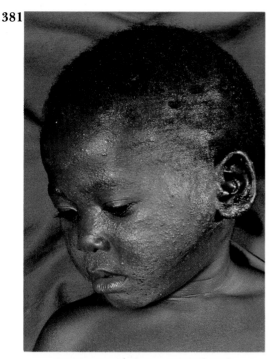

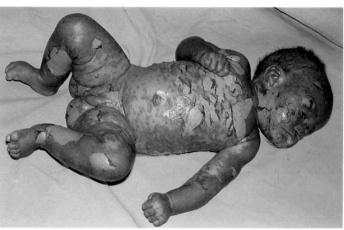

382 A four month old child on prophylactic treatment (a combination of isoniazid and thiacetazone) since the age of 1 month, because the mother had tuberculosis. Six weeks later the child developed Stevens-Johnson syndrome. Both the mother and child were infected with HIV.

381 A 3-year-old patient with AIDS who developed a drug reaction (erythroderma) to treatment (rifampicin, streptomycin, isoniazid-thiacetazone) given for pulmonary tuberculosis.

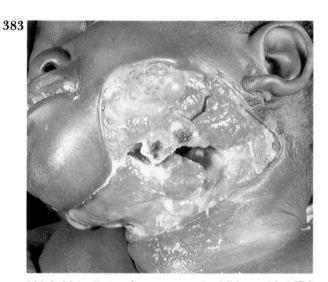

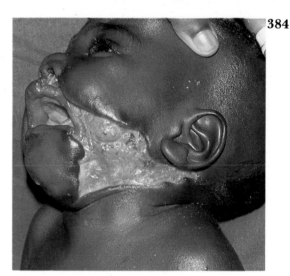

383 & 384 **Extensive cancrum** in children with AIDS.

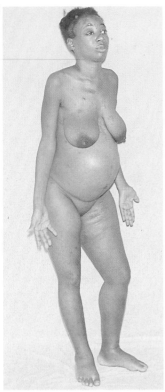

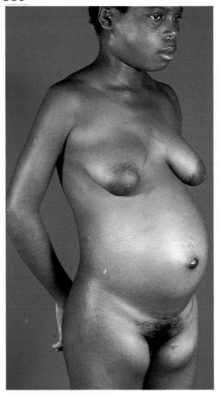

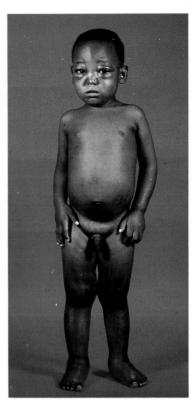

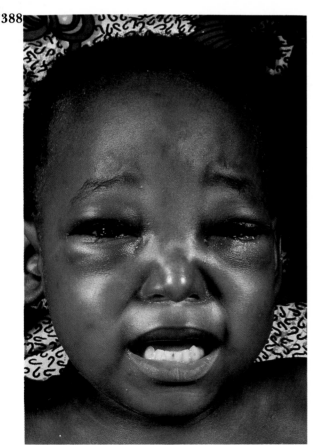

385 A pregnant woman with AAKS involving the left leg and multiple plaques on her trunk and face. She had a stillborn baby. Pregnancy wastage is common with AIDS. Pregnancy may also accelerate disease progression.

386 A pregnant woman with AAKS. She had a few vascular nodes on her face and generalised lymphadenopathy. She had a stillbirth and died a few days after labour.

387–390 This 5-year-old patient had Kaposi's sarcoma presenting clinically as nephrotic syndrome. The illustrations show puffiness of the face, ascites with oedema of the arm, a maculo-papular dermatosis and axillary adenopathy.

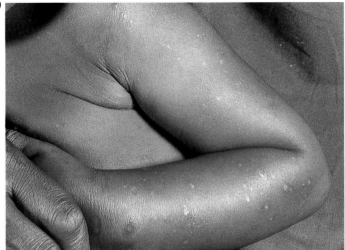

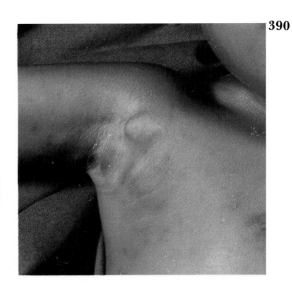

391 Identical twins born to a mother with asymptomatic HIV infection. Both were seropositive but healthy at 8 months of age.

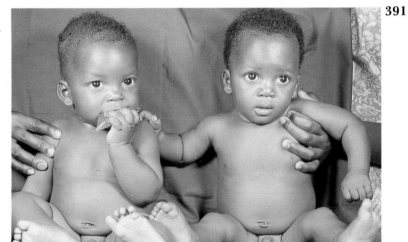

392 Identical twins born by caesarean section because of prolonged labour. The HIV status of mother at the time of caesarean section was not known. Neither the twins nor the mother were transfused. One twin was HIV infected while the other was not. The infected twin died of septicaemia and Pneumocystis carinii pneumonia at the age of eighteen months.

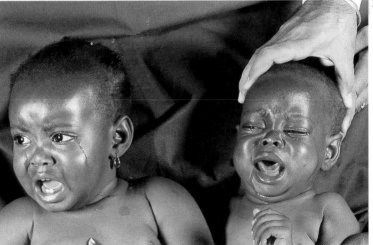

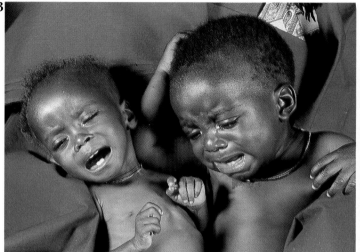

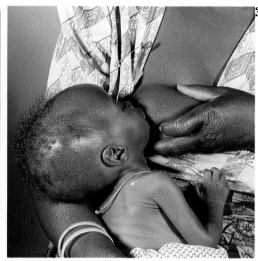

393 & 394   A one year old infant with AIDS. The mother died of AIDS. The infant was breastfed by the grandmother who had a healthy child of her own of the same age as her grandchild. The grandmother was HIV negative and continued to breastfeed till her grandson died at the age of eighteen months. The grandmother and her own child have remained seronegative for 15 months.

395

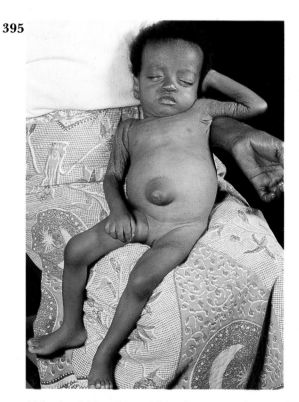

396

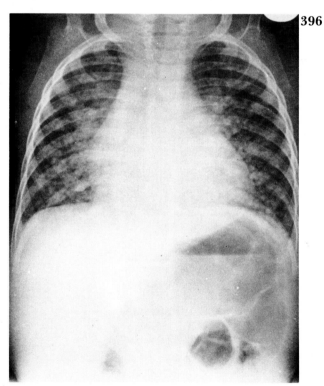

395 & 396 This child shows wasting and has circum-oral and peripheral cyanosis. The chest x-ray shows miliary pulmonary tuberculosis with mild cardiomegaly.

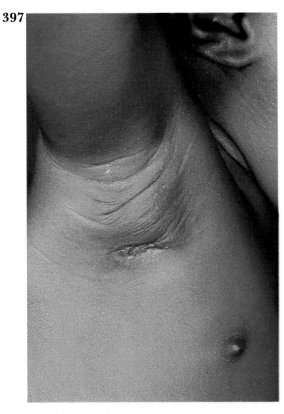

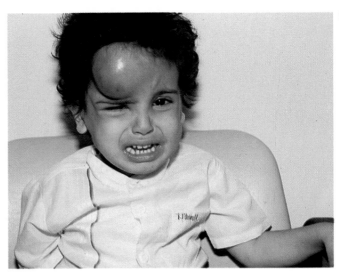

397 **Suppurative axillary adenitis** in a 6 month old HIV positive child as a result of BCG vaccination.

398 This child with a haematoma is a haemophiliac who later was found to be HIV positive by Western blot. Haemophiliacs are at risk of developing HIV infection through transfusion of unscreened blood or blood products. (By courtesy of Dr. A.W. Noorwali).

399 & 400 This 16-year-old haemophiliac had received clotting factors on several occasions. He presented with weight loss, anaemia, extensive oral candidiasis and a swelling of the left wrist with an overlying dermatophyte infection. Radiographs showed osteolytic changes in the radius forming a mass which was biopsied to give histologic diagnosis of Kaposi's sarcoma. There was a short-lived objective response to chemotherapy before the boy's final deterioration and death.

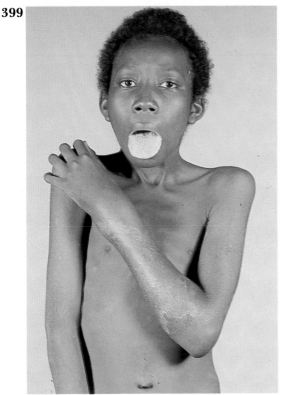

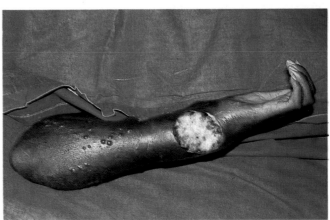

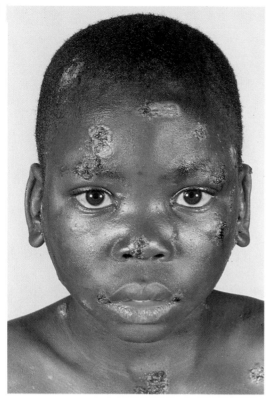

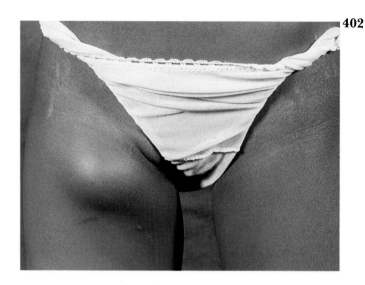

401 A 10-year-old boy with transfusion-induced ARC. He developed impetigo on face and trunk which led to ecthyma. Response to systemic antibiotics was slow.

402 & 403 This 11-year-old girl with atypical Kaposi's sarcoma and enlarged unilateral femoral lymph nodes and KS plaques on her knees. She had received a blood transfusion at the age of 8.

404 This 6-year-old boy with sickle-cell disease had received multiple blood transfusions. He developed chronic furunculosis of the scalp leading to cicatricial alopecia. His serology test was HIV positive.

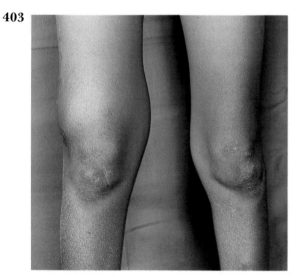

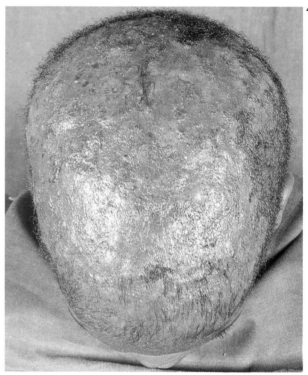

Part 3   Prevention and Health Education

Section 17: Recognised Risk Groups

Although the relative importance of risk groups in the tropics varies from country to country, risk groups include the following categories of persons:

Sexual
(a) Sexually promiscuous adults
(b) Prostitutes
(c) Homosexual and bisexual men and their partners
(d) Military personnel
(e) Truck drivers
(f) Airline personnel

Perinatal
Children born of HIV positive mothers

Blood and blood products
(a) Patients with haematological disorders who need repeated blood transfusions or blood products include:

— sickle cell disease
— thalassaemia
— haemophiliacs
(b) Intravenous drug users

Although individuals of the above groups are at higher risk, anyone who practices indiscriminate sexual activity is at risk as the disease has reached epidemic proportions. The risk of HIV-I infection from transfusion or blood products is greatly reduced but not eliminated by screening blood donors for anti-HIV-I antibody. The risk of HIV-I transmission during sexual intercourse is related to the degree of lymphopenia in the infected partner, but it can occur at any stage of HIV-I disease including the early viremic stage.

Section 18: Education for Prevention

Health education programs designed and tailored to change sexual and other risk behaviour is the most important approach for reducing the spread of human immunodeficiency virus (HIV) in the tropics and indeed, throughout the world.

Strategies for prevention and modes of transmission of this disease need to be explained to the public. This can be achieved through effective health education programmes containing simple and understandable messages. Research undertaken worldwide, as yet, has not come up with any vaccine or cure for HIV infection. Therefore, we must educate the public that prevention is the only answer.

The main objective of education for prevention is to reinforce sexual behaviour which eliminates risk of transmission of HIV.

The contents of such health education programmes should emphasize:

1. Sexual contact is the most important mode of AIDS transmission.

2. The risk increases with the number of sexual partners.

3. Restricting sexual behaviour to one partner reduces the risk.

4. The risk is reduced by using a condom.

5. AIDS can also be transmitted through blood and blood products.

6. Pregnant women who are infected with HIV can transmit the infection to their foetus.

7. Intravenous drug abuse or skin piercing techniques may transmit HIV infection.

8. There is no vaccine or cure for AIDS.

9. Prompt professional medical help should be sought by all persons who suspect that they have a sexually transmitted disease.

The above list is not in any order of priority.

Finally the specific objectives of health education programmes for prevention are to:

1. Increase knowledge in relation to above mentioned 9 key messages.

2. Correct any misconceptions and provide correct information.

3. Promote a 'healthy' attitude and belief.

4. Promote and reinforce sexual behaviour which does not involve risk of transmission.

5. Motivate change in sexual practices.

6. Increase the general level of awareness and concern regarding the existence and extent of AIDS.

Since HIV infection is virtually absent amongst primary and secondary school children, health education of this target group is the key to control of AIDS epidemic. Recognised high risk groups covered under section 17 could also be educated about transmission and prevention of HIV infection through effective utilisation of mass media.

Although mass media are commonly accepted as the best means of communication, in reality they only provide information. Communication is a two way process. The effectiveness of the mass media in changing human behaviour by providing information is not as effective as communication. The mass media, however, play an important role in sending the message to a large number of people. Educating people about prevention of HIV infection needs urgent attention.

Facilities such as television, radio, films, video-tapes, audio-tapes, newspapers, journals, posters etc. are means of reaching the masses. Both the methods of transmitting the message, and its design must take into account local cultural beliefs and attitudes, as well as the ability of the target group to understand the message. Besides providing information, the message should also motivate people to respond.

Radio broadcast messages should be designed keeping in mind the target groups. They should be short, understandable, and interesting. Similarly television "spots" should take full advantage of visual impact. Newspaper advertisements should be bold and clear. Posters should be displayed prominently in strategic places such as bus-stops, railway stations, airports, taverns, government and public buildings. Pretesting of simple messages may improve their effectiveness. Car stickers and T-shirts have also been used to stimulate public awareness.

Section 19: Protection of health workers

It should be stressed that there is no scientific reason for health personnel to be excused from delivering care to patients with AIDS.

The following precautions apply to all categories of infected persons including asymptomatic persons, patients with AIDS-related complex and patients with AIDS:

In-patient care in hospital

a. Normally, AIDS patients do not need to be isolated except in circumstances where they are at risk of acquiring hospital infection from other patients.

b. Masks should be worn by health care workers who have direct and constant contact with intubated patients requiring suction of the airways.

c. Thorough hand washing with soap and water is mandatory before and immediately after contact with patients suspected of having or known to have AIDS.

d. Gloves must be worn by those who have contact with blood, serum, tissues and any other body fluids or excretions (e.g. saliva, pus, menstrual fluid and semen). Gloves should also be worn by those coming in contact with articles or surfaces that have been contaminated by secretions and excretions. If accidental contact is made, hands should be washed immediately with soap and water.

e. If possible, goggles should be worn by health care workers in situations in which spattering with blood, blood secretions or body fluids may occur (surgeons and midwives). If the face is splashed with blood etc., the eyes and mouth should be rinsed with water to minimise the risk of infection.

f. All items visibly soiled with potentially infectious material should be considered 'infectious waste'. Contaminated linen should be put in special bags (e.g. red disposable polythene bags). Gloves should be worn when bagging the linen. All contaminated reusable linen should be decontaminated by autoclaving or boiling before washing by laundry. It is recommended that infected linen be soaked in 10% hypochlorite overnight before washing.

g. Disposable needles and syringes should never be reused.

Health care personnel who sustain any needle-prick injury should report to the Sister-in-charge of the Department and be treated according to the needle prick protocol of the Hospital Infection Control Committee. The needle prick protocol is as follows:

(1) anyone accidentally pricked with a used needle should report to the Sister-in-charge of the department.

(2) the Sister-in-charge should arrange to have the HIV-status determined, i.e. blood should be sent to the lab for anti-HIV testing, and should inform the Hospital Infection Control Committee.

(3) the individual should be advised that he/she could possibly have been infected by the needle prick and counselled appropriately.

(4) the individual should be retested for anti-HIV anti-bodies at about 3 months and again at 6 months.

(5) a history should be taken to rule out other possible means of HIV-I transmission and, if possible, a medical examination should be done to establish the current state of health of the individual.

To reduce the incidence of needle prick injuries the use of the "Anti-needle-stick device" consisting of a plastic shield is recommended.

Insert sheath through plastic, then connect to syringe. After use, resheath with hand on the opposite side of the protective plastic to avoid needle prick when resheathing.

h. Transport of Specimens
All specimens from patients should be regarded as potentially infectious. They should be collected in containers with well-fitting lids and placed in a water proof bag or container before transport. Specimens of serum from patients in outstations sent for HIV testing should be

collected preferably in a plastic container with well-fitting lid, in addition to the usual packing for transport. The serum samples may be heat inactivated (56°C, 30 min) before transportation.

i. Sterilization of Hospital Equipment

After each use lensed instruments should be cleaned physically with water and detergent/soap, then disinfected with 2% Glutaraldelyde (Cidex). Mask, mount, oral and nasopharyngeal airway Y pieces and corrugated tubing from anaesthetic machines, or ventilaters if not disposable, should be washed thoroughly and submitted for pasteurization, (70 - 80°C for at least 30 minutes) after each use. Endotracheal tubes should be preferably disposable. If not they should be sterilized before each use.

Laryngoscope blades should be replaced with a sterile blade after each use. There should be a one-way flow of instruments from the clean anaesthetists trolley to the patient and finally to a 'dirty' receiving trolley.

j. Operating Theatre

Operating theatre personnel should be informed if a known HIV positive patient is to undergo surgery, in order that special precautions can be taken in such cases. However, all patients sent to operating theatre for surgery should be considered potentially infectious especially emergency cases where the HIV status is not known. Routine sterilization and disinfection procedures of instruments and operating table before each use, should be sufficient to inactivate the HIV and prevent transmission of infection. All instruments used must be precleaned with detergents and water before disinfection and sterilisation.

Attendance at O.P.D.

The guidelines for in-patient care apply equally to out patients.

Dental Care

In addition to the guidelines already mentioned glass or stainless steel cups should be used for mouth wash and boiled for at least 20 minutes before each use.

Necropsy Mortuary Procedures

The number of people in the necropsy room should be kept to a minimum. Gowns, gloves and boots should be used. 70% ethanol, 2% glutaraldelyde and sodium hypochlorite solution, 10,000 parts per million are effective in disinfecting heavily contaminated surfaces and instruments. For floors and benches, sodium hypochlorite solution 10,000 ppm should be used. Body fluids and faeces should be decontaminated. All necropsy attendants should take care while handling sharp instruments and sharp pieces of bone so as not to prick themselves.

Histopathological Procedures

All specimens should be regarded as potentially infectious. If possible they should be sent to the laboratory in a fixative solution.

Precautions in the laboratory

In addition to guidelines mentioned above mouth pipetting should not be done. Instead, mechanical pipetting devices should be used. Care should be taken to prevent aerosol production. Laboratory work surfaces should be decontaminated with a freshly prepared solution of sodium hypochlorite 10,000 ppm following any spill and at the end of each day. This reagent should be prepared in each laboratory on a daily basis.

405 Wearing gloves is essential while performing venepuncture.

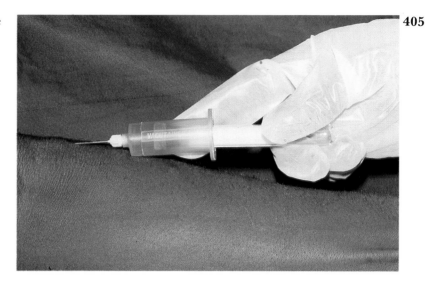

406 Hypodermic needle device for the safe disposal of needles.

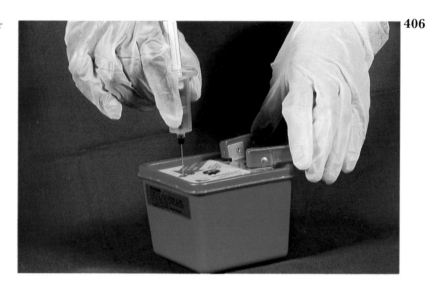

407 Improvised needle guard to prevent accidental needle stick injury to medical personnel. The needle should be resheathed through a plastic guard, eg the top of an ice-cream cup.

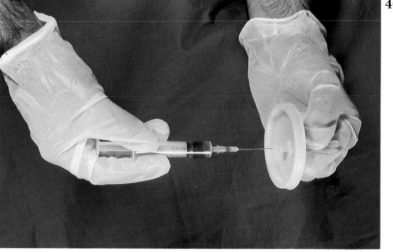

Section 20: Counselling

In the seven years since AIDS was recognised, the epidemic has affected almost all aspects of society. These include families, schools, communities, businesses and governments. Since AIDS is associated with sex, blood, drugs and death, it evokes basic human fears and inhibitions. As a result people known to be infected with HIV have been discriminated against, have lost jobs, homes and families.

Counselling is a technique by which people are assisted in helping themselves to cope with their illness, transmission of infectious agent, the psycho-social aspects and mortality. Counselling is an integral component of management of individuals infected with HIV. The technique and its context needs to be developed de novo in each country based upon the prevailing socio-cultural factors. It engenders more compassion, intelligence, selflessness and integrity on the part of health professionals.

Counselling should include:

1. Information about the patient's HIV status. The approach may be more directive for the less educated and less directive for the more educated individuals. Counsellors must allow time for the shock to sink or for emotional 'ventilation'.

2. Factual information about HIV related to its symptoms, risk of transmission, treatment and natural history.

3. The patient's concept of his or her illness.

4. Advice about change of sexual behaviour. Emphasis is placed on continuing monogamous relationship (if individual is married and both are seropositive) or abstinence (if individual is single).

5. Adjustments to be made within the family including not having any more children.

6. Support to reduce anxiety and health-damaging behaviour. Social support groups have proved to be particularly helpful in most countries and the individual should be motivated to join them.

7. Discuss and if required provide information regarding religious counselling.

The common reactions encountered during the initial and subsequent counselling are:

Denial.
A common expression encountered is "I do not believe that I have this virus. Can my blood be tested again". Repeating factual information at this stage is helpful.

Seek alternative medical opinion, including "traditional healers".
In most societies in the tropics, the traditional healers are closer to the community than the hospital based counsellors. The counselling skills of traditional healers can be recruited.

Fear or anger towards one's community or medical personnel.
Fear is manifested in form of sleepless nights, derealisation, fear of loss of weight, or diarrhoea and other symptoms associated with the virus and may not subside. Anger is generally directed towards his/her sexual partner(s). Such feelings in some individuals may lead to self-imposed isolation.

Bargaining, depression, revenge and suicide.
Some individuals ask whether they still have to follow the precautions and restrictions told to them at the first counselling session. Here the general principle is of reluctance to accept reality. Feelings of helplessness and hopelessness are commonly encountered.

Acceptance of disease.
Almost all individuals eventually accept the nature of their illness and its consequences ranging from mainly adaptive to a few maladaptive accepting behaviours.

The following situations may complicate the counselling process:

A person intending to get married.
In such a situation the sexual partner is tested and both are counselled on the basis of the results.

Married couple where only one partner is infected.
The counsellor should be careful to encourage

the couple to stay together, although the risk of transmission is explained.

Childless couple.
Most societies in the tropics are children oriented and the counsellors should carefully advise against having any children.

Pregnant patient.
Chances of in utero transmission of infection to the baby are explained and option is provided to terminate or continue with the pregnancy.

Children of parents with AIDS/ARC.
When an individual infected with HIV wishes that his grown-up children should know about the nature of his illness, the counsellor provides factual information to his/her children.

Counselling helps to achieve the following:

Behavioural changes to reduce transmission of HIV to others.

Enhances coping skills whereby the individual learns to live with the reality of HIV infection making necessary life style changes to avoid risk factors and plan his/her life purposefully.

Promotion of decision-making especially related to family problems, job situation and plans for the future.

A new concept of home care management and counselling of terminally ill patients is being tried in some countries. It is hoped that this concept will help to decongest the hospitals and provide a dignified home environment.

Index

AAKS *see* Kaposi's sarcoma, atypical African (AAKS)
Abscesses, subcutaneous 96
Acne, cystic, ARC 34
Adenitis
   axillary, childhood 115
   tuberculous 97
Adult AIDS, definition 15-16
AIDS
   CDC/WHO definition 15-16
   historical aspects 8
   immunology 10-11
   incidence/prevalence 8
   transmission 8, 117-18
   see also Paediatric AIDS
AIDS-related complex (ARC) 14, 55-7
   differential diagnosis 55
   features 55
Alopecia, furunculosis, childhood 116
Anti-globulin ELISA tests 11
Aorta, adventitia, AAKS 79
Arthritis, septic 96, 102

B-cell lymphomas 107
B-cells, polyclonal activation 11
Balanitis 26, 28
Balanoposthitis, candidal, recurrent 28
Black hairy tongue 48, 49, 57
Breast feeding, and HIV infection 108
Breast sepsis 97
Bullous dermatosis 41

Cancrum 101
   childhood 111
Candidiasis
   buccal 33
   cutaneous 47
   generalised 29, 47
   see also Oral candidiasis
Chancre, penile 19
Chancroid 18-21
   HIV-related 20, 21
   necrotic 20, 21, 22
   phagedenic 20, 21
Colon, AAKS 76
Condylomata acuminata 18, 23-6
Conjunctiva, AAKS 82
Counselling 122-3
Cryptosporidiosis, slim disease 88, 89
Cutaneous sepsis 97
Cytokines, T4 cell depletion 10
Cytotoxic antibodies, T4 cell depletion 10

Dementia 105
Dermatophyte infection 43-5
Drug eruptions
   ARC 34-8
   childhood 111

Ecthyma
   furunculosis, ARC 97
   impetigo 116
Eczema, flexural, ARC 54
ELISA tests 11
Enteropathic AIDS 88-90
Epidemiology 13
Epstein-Barr virus, hairy leucoplakia 49, 55
Erythroderma 54
   psoriatic 54
Eyelids, AAKS 81, 82

Face, nodular AAKS 66, 67
Fasciitis, necrotising 96, 103
Fauces, anterior pillars
   erythema 55, 56
   hyperaemia 56
Feet
   lymphoedema 58
   ulcers 99, 100
Fixed drug eruption 34, 35, 36
Foreign bodies, inhaled 96
Fournier's gangrene 96, 100
Frontal lobe release signs 105
Fungal infection, pulmonary 96
Furunculosis
   alopecia, childhood 116
   ecthyma, ARC 97

Gangrene 96, 100
Gastrointestinal tract, AAKS 70, 76, 80
Genitalia, oedema, AAKS 63, 64
Gingiva, AAKS 67, 68, 70, 71
Goitre, AAKS 72
Groin, AAKS plaques 63

Hair changes 53
   childhood 110
Hairy leucoplakia, tongue 49, 55
Hand, endemic KS 85, 86
Hard palate
   AAKS plaques 66, 68, 70, 71
   patchy erythema 56
Health workers, protection 119-21
Herpes genitalis 18, 26-8, 28, 51
Herpes labialis 48, 49
Herpes simplex 57
   childhood 109
Herpes zoster 28, 29-34, 62
   childhood 109
   keloids 31, 33
   ophthalmic 31
HIV-I 8, 9
   proteins 10
   transmission 13, 117-18
HIV-II 9
   epidemiology 13

HIV-related disease 14-15
  clinical features 14
  progression 14
Hospital admissions 13
HTLV-III 8, 9
HTLV-IV 9
Hypersensitivity, skin tests 12

IgM anti-HIV antibodies 12
Ileo-ileal intussusception, AAKS nodules 76
Immunodeficiency 14
Impetigo, ecthyma 116
Infants, seropositive mothers 107-8
Intertrigo, candidal 51
Isospora belli, slim disease 88

Kaposi's sarcoma (KS) 58-87
Kaposi's sarcoma, atypical African (AAKS) 53, 56, 58,
    107
  childhood 116
  confluent skin lesions 81
  differential diagnosis 58
  endemic KS differences 58
  histology 77
  lymphadenopathy 58-61
  multisystem involvement 77
  oral lesions 73, 74
  pigmentation changes 53
  thrush 71
Kaposi's sarcoma (KS), endemic 58, 87
  AAKS differences 58
  chemotherapy response 84-5
  florid tumours 83

Labour 97
Laprotomy wounds 103, 104
Lateral rectus muscle, paralysis 106
LAV 8, 9
LAV-2 9
Legs, oedema, AAKS 63
Leishmaniasis, American, cutaneous 54
Lentiviruses (slow viruses) 9
Leucopenia 55
  drug-induced 55
Leucoplakia
  debilitation associated 55
  hairy tongue 49, 55
Lobar pneumonia 91
Lungs
  AAKS 77, 78-9, 93, 94, 95
  carcinoma 96
Lymph nodes, KS 78
Lymphadenopathy
  AAKS 58-61
  tuberculous 58
  see also Persistent generalised lymphadenopathy (PGL)
Lymphogranuloma venereum 18, 22, 103
Lymphoid interstitial pneumonia 96

Maculo-papular eruptions 40-2, 88
Meningitis 106
Molluscum contagiosum 29, 50-1, 57
  genital, ARC 25

Mycosis fungoides 58
Myelopathy 105

Nail folds, lymphoedema 52
Nails
  discoloration 51-2
  pitting 52
Nephrotic syndrome, childhood KS 112
Neuralgia, herpetic 31, 33
Neurological disease, pre-AIDS 106
Neuropathy 105
Non-Hodgkin's lymphoma 107

Occipital lymph nodes, AAKS 60
Onycholysis 52
Oral candidiasis 48-9, 55, 57
  AAKS nodules 71, 73, 74-5
  slim disease 88
Osteomyelitis, femoral 100

Paediatric AIDS 107-16
  definition 16
  general immunisation 108
  transfusion-induced 108, 115, 116
Palmar nodules, AAKS 69
Pancreas, AAKS 80
Papular dermatoses 29, 40-2, 88, 89
  AAKS 83
  childhood 110
  slim disease 89
Pellagra dermatitis 47
  slim disease 88, 90
Pelvic inflammatory disease (PID) 96, 97
Penis, 'saxophone', AAKS 64
Perianal fistula 102
Perianal infection 100
Peritoneum, AAKS 80
Peritonitis 103, 104
Persistent generalised lymphadenopathy (PGL) 16-17
  fauces, hyperaemia/ erythema 56
Pigmentation changes 49, 51-3
Pigmented plaques, AAKS 69
Pinna, AAKS nodules 69
Plane warts, ARC 53
Plaques, AAKS 60-5, 67-75
Pleural effusions 92
  AAKS 93
Pneumocystis carinii pneumonia 91, 113
Pneumonia, lymphoid interstitial 96
Porphyria cutanea tarda 57
Pregnancy 97
  AAKS 112
Prevention, education 117-18
Psoriasis 28, 29, 44-6, 52
  erythrodermic 54
Pulmonary trunk, adventitia, AAKS 79
Pyomyositis, recurrent 102

Quantum spectrophotometer, ELISA tests 11

Retinitis 105
Reverse transcriptase, HIV replication 9
Risk groups 117

Scrofuloderma 101
Seborrhoeic dermatitis 28, 29, 38-40, 51
   ARC 38
Sepsis 96-104
   childhood 113
Sexual practices, AIDS prevention 117-18
Sexually transmitted diseases (STDs) 18-28
Slim disease 88-90
   differential diagnosis 88
Stevens-Johnson syndrome 37, 38, 96, 111
Stillbirth 112
Stomach, AAKS nodules 76
Subconjunctival haemorrhages, AAKS 67
Submandibular lymphadenopathy, AAKS 60
Surgical sepsis 96, 102, 104
Syncytia formation, T4 cell depletion 10
Syphilides, relapsing papular/papulosquamous 19
Syphilis, oral 18

T-helper (T4) lymphocytes
   depletion 10-11
   HIV infection 9
Thighs, AAKS plaques 63, 64
Thrush, AAKS 71

Tinea corporis 29, 49, 57, 110
Tinea imbricata, annular lesions 43
Tissue necrosis 101
Tongue
   AAKS 74
   black hairy 48, 49, 57
   hairy leucoplakia 49, 55
   pigmented filiform lesions 48, 49
Tonsils, hypertrophy 16, 17
   AAKS 72
   PGL 56
Tracheo-oesophageal fistula, children 96
Tropical ulcers 96, 99, 100
Tuberculosis
   miliary 92
   pleural effusions 92
   pulmonary 92, 96
      AAKS association 73
      childhood 114
Twins, HIV seropositive 113

Western blot, HIV antibodies 10, 12
Wounds, open 102, 103, 104